Wine

as

Food and Medicine

Wine

as

Food and Medicine

By
SALVATORE P. LUCIA, A.B., M.D., Sc.D., F.A.C.P.
Professor of Medicine,
University of California School of Medicine

New York • THE BLAKISTON COMPANY, INC. • Toronto

LIBRARY OF CONGRESS CATALOG CARD NO. 54–7397

PRINTED IN THE UNITED STATES OF AMERICA
AT THE COUNTRY LIFE PRESS, GARDEN CITY, N.Y.

Preface

As a food and medicine, wine is important in the life of man. It is significant not only because of the intricate chemistry of the grape (a botanical and biological phenomenon) but also because of the complex nature of the finished product. Wine is the most ancient dietary beverage and the most important medicinal agent in continuous use throughout the history of mankind.

Before the era of Pasteur, scientific enquiries into the dietary and medicinal uses of wine were practically non-existent, yet a tremendous reference literature had accumulated on the empirical uses of wine as a nutritional and medicinal agent. The ancient Greek physicians were divided into two groups, those who used wine therapeutically and those who did not. Hippocrates was among the first to advocate the artful use of wine in the healing of the sick. In the twenty-five hundred years since his time, the prescription of wine has swung from universal use to almost complete prohibition and back again. There has been a most imposing procession of advocates of wine as food and medicine— Erasistratus, Asclepiades, Horace, Celsus, Columella, Pliny, Athenaeus, Dioscorides, and Galen, among the ancients; Oribasius, Aëtius, Alexander of Tralles, Paul of Aegina, Rhazes, Avicenna, Maimonides, Arnald of Villanova and Guy de Chauliac during the Middle Ages. In the Bible, Paul advises Timothy, "Drink no longer water, but use a little wine for thy stomach's sake and thine often infirmities." Pasteur has written: "Wine is the most healthful and the most hygienic of beverages." Actually, few other substances available to man have been as widely recommended for their curative powers as have wines.

Subsequent to the work of Pasteur, much of value was recorded concerning the nutritional and medicinal properties of the fermented juice of the grape. This literature was relatively insignificant when compared with the voluminous modern literature on the technology of the production of wine, its chemistry, and the potential physiologic effects of wine, which followed the definition of the science of physiologic chemistry and the application of its finer techniques to the study of living processes. It indicates that the contemplation of wine is important from every possible aspect of human interest—historic, social, biologic, psychologic, and medical. No one, not even the prohibitionist, can afford to ignore the importance of wine.

Unfortunately, an entire generation of physicians in the United States lost touch with the medical lore of wine following the first World War. Prohibition proved to be a costly experiment. Many physicians were not only denied the opportunity to comprehend the therapeutic values of a well-tried agent, but they were conditioned to the uncritical acceptance of the latest pharmaceutical development, using it avidly for a time, and then discarding it completely—only to take over the next product heralded as a panacea. There is much more logic in using an agent that has proved successful for centuries and is known to be harmless to the human organism. There are many investigators who are devoting their energies to exploring complex medicinal agents, found to be useful empirically, in an attempt to determine the nature of the active principles which make them effective. With adequate techniques this approach could be applied profitably to the study of wine.

In recent years there has developed within the medical profession a demand for an evaluation of wine as a medicinal agent, and for the separation of fact from folklore. There has been expressed a desire for an impartial study and analysis of those elements which can be scientifically measured. We can say that these desires have been appreciated and that active research is in process on many phases of the scientific evaluation of wine both pharmacodynamically and physiologically.

In the wild scramble for therapeutic specificity, little thought has been given to the psychotherapeutic effects of the simple adjuvants to living that make life worth while. No one can deny that a remedy, in order to be successful, must induce psychologic effects, despite their immeasurability. On the other hand, no remedy for an organic illness can be successful if it produces only a psychologic effect. Many of the imputed medicinal effects of vinous products are due to the fact that psychologically wine is acceptable and physiologic. Furthermore, partaking of wine offers an opportunity for psychic rest and release from the pressures of the day; it also provides time for recovery from mental fatigue so that the psyche may be better able to cope with our frenetic mode of living.

This text deals with wine as a food and a medicine. In regard to the former, reference to a significant bibliography perhaps is all that is necessary. For the latter, an impressive, prodigious and scattered bibliography is available for those who wish to consult it. This book is offered as a *vade mecum* to those who are unprejudiced in their search for that which makes men desire to live against odds often insurmountable.

In the discussion of the chemistry of wine will be found a simple catalogue of those elements which can be readily defined. It is our opinion that the effect of wine as an adjuvant to the dietary, the psychologic, and the vital corporeal functions is more than the effect of alcohol. No one would assume that an aqueous solution of alcohol would be an appropriate or acceptable accompaniment to a fine meal. Nor would one expect to obtain from an aqueous solution of alcohol those yet-to-be-defined delicate sympathomimetic reactions of the diverse aldehydic complexes of wine. Perhaps there is a relationship between the structure of some of the chemical compounds found in so kaleidoscopic a mixture as wine and the infinite variety of psychic reactions induced by wine. These present a challenge to future research. Who knows what elements influence Nepenthe? Superficially the physiologic effects of wine are those of ethyl alcohol, but with more careful analyses of the biologic and psychologic reactions it induces, one realizes that elements other than alcohol play singular and important rôles.

The author takes this opportunity to express his thanks to Miss Carolyn B. Dingley and Miss Bertha Landauer for able bibliographic assistance; to Professor Maynard A. Amerine for criticism and guidance in the chapter on the Chemistry of Wine; to Professor Hamilton H. Anderson for notes and advice on certain pharmacologic aspects of wine; and to his many colleagues, members of the Society of Medical Friends of Wine for information and anecdotes concerning their respective specialties; to Mrs. Kathleen Doyle, appreciation and thanks for the part she played in the compilation of the data necessary for the conversion of the material into its present form; to Miss Dorothy Lowe for editorial assistance, for the skillful use of the Wine Library and Bibliographic Files on the medical uses of wine at the University of California School of Medicine, and for the countless hours she spent in ferreting out recondite statements buried in volumes devoid of indices; and lastly to my many colleagues on the faculty of the School of Medicine, who pressed me to record these data concerning a subject for which I have great warmth and fondness, despite my reluctance to do so in the face of an overburdened schedule. What interest the book may create has not been anticipated; what errors the text may contain are those of the author solely; and what help it may be to those who consult it will be compensation enough for having written it.

SALVATORE P. LUCIA

December, 1953   *San Francisco*

Contents

I. *The Chemistry of Wine*

Wine is a chemically complex product of the naturally fermented juice of the grape. The constituents responsible for its distinctive characteristics are alcohols, aldehydes, fixed and volatile acids, carbon dioxide, nitrogenous compounds, inorganic constituents, coloring matter, tannins, esters, sugars, pectin, vitamins, and aroma-producing substances. The physiologic effects of wine can be predicted if the chemistry and the biologic reactions of its individual constitutents are understood.

Alcohols

Physiologically and quantitatively the most important constituent of wine, aside from water, is alcohol—a product of the fermentation of the sugars contained within the grape. Sugars are formed in the foliage of the vine and translocated to the grapes during the maturation of the fruit. The amount of sugar in the mature grape varies according to the type of grape, the quantity of sunshine it receives, the character of the soil in which it grows, and the climatic conditions to which the vine is exposed during its periods of growth and dormancy. In the process of fermentation, the sugars, dextrose and levulose, are converted by a complex series of biochemical reactions into ethyl alcohol, carbonic acid, and small quantities of other important organic compounds. Due to the greater avidity with which

11

dextrose is attacked and broken down by the action of most yeasts, the sugar which remains in wine after fermentation is chiefly levulose. The proportion between dextrose and levulose differs from one wine to another and depends to some extent upon the agents of fermentation, the point at which fermentation may be stopped, and the amount of sugar originally present in the must. In any case, the amount of reducible sugar remaining in the finished wine is characteristic of the type of wine. Decomposition of the sugars takes place through the agency of *Saccharomyces cerevisiae* var. *ellipsoideus,* of which various vinous strains are known. Yeasts capable of fermenting sugars exist everywhere in nature and in many cases are present in sufficient quantity on the surface of the grapes to provide for normal alcoholic fermentation. For uniform results under all conditions and particularly under unfavorable climatic conditions, it has been found desirable to cultivate and add certain strains of yeast to the crushed grapes in order to obtain a better end-product. The ratio of sugar to alcohol can be predicted roughly by the use of the Gay-Lussac equation, namely, that one molecule of dextrose or levulose will yield two molecules each of ethyl alcohol and carbon dioxide.

In addition to ethyl alcohol, wine also contains traces of higher alcohols. Among these are isopropyl, isobutyl, iso-amyl, hexyl, heptyl, and nonyl, which are collectively called "fusel oils," and are mainly derived from the deamination of amino acids. When the higher alcohols occur in appreciable amounts they may give the wine an unpleasant taste. The most important polyhydric alcohol of wine is glycerol (glycerine), and it is found in appreciable traces in all wines, especially in those derived from grapes containing a high sugar content, or from grapes which have been hosts to the *Botrytis cinerea* mold during the ripening process. The amount of glycerol in wine averages from 7 to 12 per cent of the alcohol content and rarely exceeds 16 per cent. Similar compounds which appear in minute quantities in wine are

2, 3-butyleneglycol and acetylmetholcarbinol. Mannitol is found only in "sick" wines.

Methyl alcohol is not an important product of the fermentation of sugar but is derived mainly from the hydrolysis of pectins. Red wines, which are fermented on the skins, therefore may contain more methyl alcohol than white wines, but the amount present is negligible and in such small concentrations it produces no untoward physiologic effects.

Aldehydes

Aldehydes are dehydrogenated alcohols and are formed when alcohol is oxidized without loss of carbon. For every alcohol there is a corresponding aldehyde. The simplest aldehyde, formaldehyde, appears in wine in such small traces that it can be completely disregarded as a natural component. Acetaldehyde is present in minute quantities in all wines, and particularly in those which have been in contact with oxygen over a long period of time. Wines that have been aerated contain increased amounts of acetaldehyde, which imparts to them a characteristic vapid odor. All wines which have been treated with sulfur dioxide contain a bisulfite-aldehyde complex and possess less of the objectionable sulfurous or vapid odor of sulfur dioxide or acetaldehyde and also less of the antiseptic property of an equivalent amount of sulfur dioxide. These changes are due to the chemical combination of the sulfur dioxide with the reactive constituents of the wine.

Acids

Among the acids contained in wine are those which are already found in grapes such as tartaric, malic, citric, phosphoric, and tannic; and those which are produced during or after alcoholic fermentation such as carbonic, formic, acetic, lactic and succinic. In addition, sulfurous and sulfuric acids are both present in traces when sulfur dioxide has been used in the preparation of the wine. Wine also contains traces of the fatty acid series such as propionic, butyric, valeric, caproic, caprylic and particularly oenanthic, probably as a result of bacterial activity and predominantly in the esterified form. The "oenanthic ether" or ester, from the Greek, "grape bloom" exists mainly as ethyl *n*-heptylate (ethyl enanthate). The organoleptic substances closely allied to "oenanthic ether" include the ethyl esters of capric, caproic, caprylic and pelargonic acids, as well as amyl caproate and isoamyl butyrate and other esters.

The most characteristic acid of wine is the dibasic tartaric acid. Of its six known varieties, only two, the more common dextrotartaric and the optically inactive racemic tartaric acid, are universally present in wine. The tartrates, mostly in the form of potassium acid tartrate, occur in natural wines up to 5 grams per liter. The quantity of free acid present is dependent upon the pH of the wine. The amount of free tartaric acid compared to the acid salt and salts is usually higher in dry white table wines than in dry red table wines. During fermentation and storage of the wine, the potassium acid tartrate present in the musts becomes partially separated from the wine in a crystalline form. The extent to which this occurs depends largely upon changes of temperature and the concentration of alcohol. In any event, the total tartrate content of the finished product represents only a fraction of the total nonvolatile acids of the wine.

The amount of malic acid present in wine depends upon the ripeness of the grapes and the way the wine develops following fermentation. During this period, malic acid may be partially or wholly converted by bacterial action into carbon dioxide and lactic acid. The time required for the conversion of malic acid varies with the pH of the wine, its temperature, and the type and amount of the microflora present. Wines of high pH value may show decomposition of malic acid during the primary fermentation, while wines of low pH values may not undergo malo-lactic fermentation until the temperature rises in the summer of the year following the primary fermentation. Even after a wine is bottled, malic acid may be transformed into lactic acid and carbon dioxide, and thus produce a gassy wine. Lactic acid, which is never found in the juice of fresh grapes, is ordinarily considered a nonvolatile acid, even though it may behave in part like a volatile acid when subjected to steam. Where the original malic acid content is high and the malolactic fermentation more or less complete, lactic acid may be the dominant acid in the finished wine.

Citric acid, a normal constituent of wine, is found in the finished natural product in concentrations of not more than 500 milligrams per liter. Greater amounts indicate an admixture with wine of fruits other than grapes, or the addition of citric acid during vinification. Succinic acid, which develops during fermentation, is always present in natural wine in small quantities. The probable source material is glutamic acid. It may also be a by-product of the metabolic action of yeast on sugars during alcoholic fermentation. The sulfuric and sulfurous acids and the sulfates present in wine are traceable to the sulfurous acid which is added to inhibit oxidation and bacterial contamination while the wine is being stabilized and prepared for storage.

In modern wine chemistry, the development and fining of wine must be considered in the light of the reduction-oxidation potentials of the fermented grape juice. This phenomenon is expressed as the "redox-potential" and can be measured electrometrically. It is designated in terms of rH (analogous to pH) ; a value over 25 is considered as oxidant and one under 15 as reductant. Sulfur dioxide, a strong reducing agent, so drastically decreases the rH value of musts that only "sulfite yeasts" can grow normally in musts thus treated. Ultimately, the flavor of a wine is affected by the chemical reactions expressed in the "redox-potential" equilibrium. In recent years the use of sulfur dioxide as an inhibitor of oxidation and contamination has been replaced to some extent by the technique of germ-proof filtering which removes almost all microorganisms, particularly the yeast cells. The wine which passes through these filters is thus rendered practically sterile. The disadvantage of the so-called germ-proof filtering technique is that occasionally it interferes with malo-lactic fermentation.

While hydrogen sulfide is present only accidentally in finished wines, compounds of phosphoric acid, which are permanent natural ingredients, are always found—in fact, without their presence alcoholic fermentation cannot take place. The derivatives of phosphoric acid and their enzymes are more abundant in red than in white wines. Since boron is universally present in soil, almost all wines contain traces of boric acid in the form of its hydrate; the quantity may amount to as much as 50 milligrams per liter. Salicylic acid, derived from the salicylates of the grape stalk, is found in many wines in the form of esters, but in trace quantities only (less than 1 milligram per liter). Appreciable traces of benzoic and silicic acids occur in normal healthy wines in concentrations up to 7 milligrams and 50 milligrams per liter, respectively.

Finally, any excess acidity apparent to the taste is due to the amount of tartaric, citric, lactic, malic, succinic and volatile acids present, which influence the ultimate pH of the wine. The presence of any considerable amount of acetic acid is evidence that a wine is unsound; the presence of appreciable amounts of malic acid indicates that the wine was made from underripe grapes; and the absence of tartaric acid demonstrates that probably calcium was added to the wine.

The amount of *volatile acid* in healthy natural wines varies from about 0.2 to 1.2 grams per liter. The presence of larger quantities indicates that the wines are undergoing undesirable oxidative changes. The volatile acidity should not be more than 0.11 per cent in a dry white table wine, and 0.12 per cent in a red table wine. Among the volatile acids of wine, acetic acid heads the list in importance. It appears both as a by-product of fermentation and as an ester in the form of ethyl acetate. Young wines are often so rich in acetic acid that they possess the typical odor of acetate ester, and it has been demonstrated that the ethyl acetate formed by the acetic acid bacteria rather than the acetic acid itself produces the objectionable sharp taste of vinegary wine.

Very small amounts of the fatty acids (formic, propionic, butyric, valeric, and the higher acids, caproic, caprylic and capric, as well as oleic and myristic) are found in wines. In part they are bound to bases and in part esterified with alcohol and, to a very small extent, with glycerol. At least some wines contain caproic, caprylic and capric acids. Butyric and valeric acids are normal constituents of all wines—approximately 10 to 20 milligrams per liter each. Small quantities of glyceric esters of oleic and myristic acids, mainly originating from the fat of the yeast, have been reported in wines. Oenanthic acid occurs only in combination with alcohol as oenanthic ester. It is probably formed during the process of fermentation.

Carbon Dioxide

According to the Gay-Lussac equation, the molecular amount of carbon dioxide formed during primary fermentation is approximately the same as that of ethyl alcohol. The gas so formed is lost by volatilization. Later, small amounts may be produced in bottle during the malo-lactic fermentation of malic acid. Wines rich in alcohol contain more natural carbon dioxide than weak wines. Many of the fine, light white table wines of the world are prepared, stored, and marketed in such a manner that their natural carbon dioxide content is preserved. This gives them a delicate *pétillance* and enhances their quality and organoleptic character. On the other hand, carbon dioxide may be added to any wine in order to embellish it. Champagnization is accomplished by imprisoning the carbon dioxide formed by the selective fermentation of added sugar or by entrapping the gas in the wine under conditions of controlled temperature and pressure.

Nitrogen Compounds

The nitrogen compounds in *wine musts* vary from 300 to 1000 milligrams per liter, about 50 to 150 milligrams being in the ammoniacal form. The average *wine* seldom contains less than 100 milligrams per liter; better wines, as well as those which have been left on the yeast for a longer period of time, may contain as much as 900 milligrams per liter. It is assumed that wines containing less than 70 milligrams of nitrogen per liter have suffered from dilution.

Most of the organic nitrogen of wines is present as amino acids, peptides, and purines, with but small traces in the form of whole protein. Seven different fractions of nitrogen compounds have been identified in the fresh musts of white wines. These are, in the order of their magnitude: (*1*) *amino acid nitrogen* (alanine, valine, tyrosine, leucine, proline, serine, threonine, glutamic acid, aspartic acid, and phenylalanine) including nitrogen obtained from some dipeptides; (*2*) *phosphotungstic nitrogen,* including that obtained from tripeptides, tetrapeptides, diamino acids, *i.e.,* arginine and lysine, heterocyclic acids, *i.e.,* histidine and proline, and traces of purines and pyrimidines. Among the groups of lesser importance are: (*3*) *ammonia nitrogen;* (*4*) *amide nitrogen* (aspargine and glutamine); (*5*) *humin nitrogen* (tyrosine and tryptophane); (*6*) *protein nitrogen;* and (*7*) *residue nitrogen* (including compounds of unknown composition).

The nitrogen content of wine is important for the nutrition of yeasts and certain varieties of bacteria, and the production of higher alcohols during fermentation. In addition, during the processes of settling and clarification the nitrogen compounds assist in the production of clear and brilliant wines.

Extract and Mineral Substances

When wine is evaporated at 100° C., the residue is called extract. From the ashing of extract, the total quantity of inorganic substances, anionic and cationic, is obtained. The weight of ash recovered from wine varies between 1.5 and 3.5 grams per liter, or about 10 per cent of the weight of the extract. The quality of the wine, to a certain extent, is determined by its quantity of extract. Whenever the amount of extract falls below 17.5 grams per liter for white wines, and 18.5 grams per liter for red wines, such wines are referred to as "thin" and most likely have been diluted. For the sake of taste, the mineral content of white wines should exceed 1.3 grams per liter and for red wines 1.6 grams per liter. During years of scarce rainfall, the mineral content of wine is apt to be low; during periods of abundant rainfall, wines will be richer in minerals. The total quantity, however, will be conditioned by geographic location and the specific character of a given soil as a repository for minerals.

The mineral ash of wine consists of potassium, sodium, magnesium, calcium, and iron combined in phosphates, carbonates, sulfates, chlorides, and oxides, with minor traces of other mineral substances. Potassium, which accounts for about 40 per cent of the ash, is highly soluble and found closely bound to tartaric acid. Although new wines contain about 4.0 to 5.0 grams of potassium per liter, the finished product may contain less than 2.0 grams per liter because some is precipitated out as potassium acid tartrate during storage. Sodium appears in the ash in varying amounts—10 to 60 or more milligrams per liter—depending upon the richness in sodium of the particular soil. Magnesium is found in concentrations of 60 to 144 milligrams per liter. This mineral seems to act as a catalyst and without it fermentation cannot take place. Aluminum appears in trace quantities in the finished product. The amount of manganese varies greatly, its concentration averaging about 3 milligrams per liter. Boron and silicon have already been discussed as boric and silicic acids. Grapes from vines treated with arsenical pest-controlling agents usually contain some free arsenic which may be found in traces in the finished product. However, wines made from grapes not so treated may also contain traces of arsenic. The content of chlorine usually averages 20 to 80 milligrams per liter, and the amount of sodium chloride seldom exceeds 100 milligrams per liter. Wine generally contains from 0.1 to 0.2 milligrams of iodine per liter. Fluorine is frequently found in the ash but never in quantities exceeding 10 milligrams per liter.

Some minerals foreign to the grape may be present in wine because they come in contact with the vines or with the wine during fermentation. Among these are lead, which remains on the vines and grapes after they have been sprayed with lead preparations; copper and zinc, found in trace quantities when wine has been kept in vessels containing these minerals; and, finally, iron which may appear in wine as ferrous or ferric salts depending upon the degree of oxidation. The latter, in limited quantities, is considered by some to be an important organoleptic substance.

Whatever minerals there are or whatever their source may be, the amount of such materials in wine varies considerably. In pure natural wines the quantity of ash fluctuates between 1.5 and 3.5 grams per liter, while in wines in which excessive acidity has been neutralized, the ash content will be considerably greater.

Coloring Matter

Good wines, matured by age, are never colorless. Those which are white in the beginning take on color because the air which reaches them exerts an oxidizing effect on the extractives. The color of wine is further deepened by the tannins derived from the skins, pips and stems of the grapes during fermentation, as well as by the tannin absorbed from the oak casks in which it is stored. These materials intensify the mixture of green and yellow pigmentary substances—chlorophyll, carotene and xanthophyll—which occur naturally in grapes. As the grapes ripen, the content of chlorophyll decreases and finally appears in the husks decomposed into yellowish-green, amber-yellow and brownish pigments. The yellow pigmentary substances, quercetin and quercitrin, are contained in both red and white grapes, and their wines. In addition, red wines contain oenin. Although it has not been demonstrated that chlorophyll, carotene, or xanthophyll are present in the finished wine, there is no doubt about the presence of quercetin and quercitrin.

The color of red wine is due primarily to the anthocyanin, oenin (a monoglucoside of oenidin), which is formed in the plant by the action of sunshine and translocated to the exterior cell layers of the grape. Oenin is leached out of grape skins during fermentation. The tint which a red wine finally assumes depends upon several factors: the amount of coloring matter in the wine, the pH of the wine, and the oxidation-reduction conditions which partially depend upon the content of tannin, oxygen and iron. The greater the quantity of free acid (the lower the pH), the redder the wine. Most red wines contain sufficient natural pigment so that no special fermentation procedures or treatments are needed to increase their color.

Tannins

Tannins must also be considered in connection with the ultimate color of wine. The skins and stems of grapes contain most of the tannin, which accounts for the fact that red wines, which are allowed to ferment on the skins, are richer in this substance than white wines. Tannin serves to fix pigmentary substances and it imparts to wines their characteristic astringent taste. The tannin found in white wines comes largely from the oak casks in which it is matured before bottling. Pale yellow at first, white wines become deeper in color with age. Part of this is due to the absorption of oxygen which converts tannin into a yellow or brown pigmentary substance.

Proteinaceous Substances

The nitrogenous materials of the grape are precipitated following fermentation of the must. Those proteinaceous substances which remain on the surface exposed to air are liable to oxidation as well as decomposition and the products so formed may taint the wine. Since properly-fermented white wines contain a minimum of nitrogenous materials, they remain relatively invulnerable to this source of hazard. Imperfectly fermented wines and wines made from underripe grapes are subject to change because some of the proteinaceous materials remain suspended in the wine. The proteinaceous substances of young red wines are stabilized by the presence of tannin, and in the course of aging are precipitated with the tannin and coloring matters of the wine. Chemically and physiologically, the quantity of protein in properly fermented wine is practically negligible.

Esters

Esters are compounds formed by the non-ionic reaction of acids and alcohols and many of them are responsible for the characteristic aromas and flavors of wine. Esterification of alcohols and acids in wine may be the result of chemical or biologic activity. The former is responsible mainly for the volatile odoriferous ethyl esters of low molecular weight acids, chiefly acetic, and the latter for the neutral and acid esters of fixed acids, such as tartaric and malic. The manner in which esterification is conditioned may influence the proportion of esters due to chemical activity in relation to those of biologic activity. Biologic esterification is predominantly the result of the reactions of yeasts, bacteria, enzymes, and aging in the production of wine. The highly controversial "oenanthic ether" appears as a product of wine during the aging process.

Ethyl acetate is perhaps the most abundant ester en-countered in young wine. Recent researches have indicated that, contrary to opinion, it may be an undesirable aromatic constituent. The relative amount of the volatile neutral ester (ethyl acetate) present in wine, when compared with the quantity of total esters, may be used as an indicator of the age of a sample of wine. The quantity of this ester is limited only by the bulk of water which wine contains.

When propyl, butyl, and amyl alcohols combine with acetic acid, esters are produced which possess some of the characteristics of ethyl acetate; that is, they contribute both to the flavor and the bouquet of the wine in which they are found. As acetic acid forms a series of esters with the various alcohols of wine, there is also a series of esters composed of the various acids with a given alcohol. In wine we may expect these acids always to combine with the pre-vailing alcohol, namely ethyl. The esterification of acids and alcohol is apparently facilitated and enriched by the presence of tartaric acid. Many of the fixed acid esters possess distinctive fragrances which may be highly advan-tageous to a wine. Frequently the aroma of a concentrated ester is unpleasant but, when diluted as in wine, it becomes desirable, agreeable, and reminiscent of the flavor of fruit.

Wine derives its special characteristic as a union of flavors resulting from fermentation and the production of "oenanthic esters." These have been called the "grape bloom or bouquet ethers." Although many other aromatic substances share in producing the total saporific effect, oenanthic esters are significant because without them wine as we know it would not be the important and pleasant beverage it is.

Oenanthic ester is a colorless, oily liquid which passes over in very small quantities after the distillation of large volumes of wine. It has been called "Oil of Cognac" and probably is a chemically impure mixture of various esters. It is stated that forty thousand parts of wine yield only one part of the aromatic oil. It is soluble in diluted spirit, but insoluble in water. It is believed that the characteristic odor of wine—as differentiated from that of other fermented beverages—is due in a large part to the presence of this substance.

Ethyl tartrate, the only tartaric acid ester appearing in wine, is a crystallizable but deliquescent solid body which reacts like an acid, even forming salts with bases. It cannot be distilled because it disintegrates into various products at the distillation temperature.

In addition to the esters already discussed, innumerable compound esters which further enhance the bouquet appear in wine. It is conceivable that a wine containing six alcohols and six acids might form thirty-six different esters, all of which would contribute to the flavor and the fragrance of the wine, with the predominant combinations determining the predominant aroma and taste. The "bouquet substances," some already present in the grapes, remain unchanged during fermentation, and others appear as a result of fermentation or during the aging process. The quantity of some "bouquet substances" is so negligible and their characters so unstable that their isolation has presented a great challenge to wine chemists. Among substances found in small amounts, a lipid, lecithin (260 to 290 milligrams per liter) is present in all natural wines, the red wines containing a greater quantity than the white wines. Many of the important ingredients of wine have already been accurately defined and with improvements in techniques others will be identified.

Pectic Substances

Pectic materials, soluble and colloidal, occur in grapes in varying quantities. Some of them are lost during the period of fermentation and others may be destroyed by hydrolyzing enzymes during the clarification processes. The soluble pectic materials may exert a beneficial effect on the smoothness of wines; however, they are precipitated by alcohol unless held in suspension by protective substances or some other mechanism yet to be defined.

In the hydrolysis of pectin, the pectic acid reacts like a glucoside and these materials may influence the substance of the wine. A monogalacturonic acid has been identified as one component of pectin.

Vitamins

The vitamin content of fresh grapes varies somewhat with the variety and the environmental conditions under which the grapes are grown. During the crushing and fermentation of the grape much of the easily oxidized vitamin C is lost. The vitamins originate chiefly in the plant itself but some will be derived from the wine yeasts, especially vitamin D substances, some of which have been identified as ergosterin.

Vitamin A, its pro-vitamin, and carotenoids have been identified in the edible portion of the grape. Of the vitamin B complex, thiamin, riboflavin, pyridoxin, pantothenic acid, nicotinic acid and inositol have been identified. Some flavones having the chemical and physiologic properties of rutin and some of the physical characteristics of the so-called vitamin P group occur in grapes and in wine. Grapes have been reported to be one of the richest sources of vitamin P.

In wine, the amounts of the various vitamins fluctuate markedly. Although many of the vitamins are present in wine, we must admit that the amounts of some of them are negligible or only found in trace quantities. In general, wine is not to be considered a rich source of vitamins.

II. *The Physiologic Effects of Wine*

The grape is one of the few fruits of the earth endowed by nature with a pulp containing substances of unlimited potentialities when transformed by the miracles of fermentation. The phylogenetic processes of morphology and cellular chemistry have surfeited the grape with constituents which, in the transformation following fermentation, endow the final product with distinctive and individual effects. The most pronounced physiologic effect of transformed grape juice depends upon ethyl alcohol. Under the influence of alcohol, the salivary mucous membrane is provoked to secrete directly and reflexly an abundant flow of saliva, the repercussions of which are felt in the stomach by an increase in the secretion of hydrochloric acid.[1] Gastric secretions are stimulated also by the direct administration of alcohol. If, however, the concentration of alcohol surpasses the optimum, then the albumin-coagulating action of the alcohol, the changes in osmotic pressure, and other physicochemical alterations will induce a suppression of secretion.

In discussing the influence of wine on absorption, it is advisable to deal first with the effects of alcohol in solution before referring to the other constituents of wine which impart physiologic effects, as well as endow the various vintages with their specific characteristics. It has been demonstrated experimentally that a solution of ethyl alcohol in pure water is absorbed as follows: minimal amounts in

the mouth, 20 per cent in the stomach, 10 per cent in the
upper jejunum, 50 per cent in the middle small intestine,
20 per cent in the terminal ileum,[2] none being found in the
feces.[3] Its transport into the blood, therefore, is complete
and more rapid than that of starchy foods. The level of
maximum concentration in the blood stream is reached in
from one-half to two hours, and this may be taken to signify
the period of the maximum stimulating effect. The speed
of absorption of alcohol from different wines varies according to the content of alcohol in the wine, the composition of the wine, and the time of its ingestion in relation to
meals. Fatty substances, such as cream, retard absorption
to a much greater extent than proteinaceous foods such as
meat.[4] Fat apparently exerts its effect by actually interfering
with the absorption of alcohol from the stomach, whereas
other food substances exert their specific effect by combining
with the alcohol and interfering with the rate of metabolism
of alcohol. Experimentally it has been shown that the blood
alcohol level is diminished when the amino acids, alanine
and glycine, are dissolved in the alcohol.[5] The absorption of
alcohol from wine is slower than the absorption of the same
amount of ethyl alcohol diluted in water or taken as spirit
diluted in water. The absorption of alcohol is quickened
by any factor which increases the rate of absorption or
motility of the bowel. The absorption of white wines is
more rapid than that of red wines of equal alcoholic
strength.[6] Citric, malic, tartaric, phosphoric acids, and the
higher fatty acids which are often found in wine also delay
the rate of absorption of alcohol due in part to the fact
that free fatty acids remove a large part of alcohol from
the attack of metabolic processes. This effect is further
increased when glycerol and oleic acid are given simultaneously.[7]

The laws of diffusion govern the transit of alcohol from
the blood into the tissues where the largest part of it is
metabolized. Experiments have indicated that an allowance

of 50 milliliters of alcohol taken with a meal, or 100 milliliters taken daily in any form whatever, represents the maximum amount which can be completely metabolized by the average person,[8] although Widmark[9] placed this level at 170 grams of absolute alcohol for a man weighing 70 kilograms. An excess intake leaves a residue which must be handled by the organism in a less efficient manner.[10]

Metabolically, alcohol exerts a sparing effect on carbohydrate and especially on fat by replacing these energy-forming substances of the diet. It may not spare body protein, but when added to the diet it promotes the storage and accelerates the growth of young animals subsisting on high protein diets.[11] The experiments of Atwater and Benedict have demonstrated that alcohol, energy-wise, can completely replace the nonnitrogenous dietary substances. Whether this same effect is achieved with the nitrogenous food substances depends largely upon the amount of alcohol taken, its concentration, the metabolic state, and the age of the subject. Small amounts of alcohol exert a protein-sparing effect from the very beginning. On the other hand, 100 milliliters of alcohol taken daily in lieu of fat, isodynamically, results in an increased disintegration of albumin, the effect not being apparent until the organism has become habituated to the alcohol intake. In either case, the protein-sparing effect of ingested alcohol occurs whether the alcohol balances an equivalent amount of fat or of carbohydrate in the diet.

In physiologic amounts, alcohol may deepen the respiratory excursions. It has very little effect on the healthy heart, although the pulse volume may be increased. Even large amounts of alcohol may not appreciably alter the frequency of the pulse, unless the function of the heart be altered by disease. It has been stated that the liver is the pace-maker[12] for the metabolism of alcohol, since the initial reaction in a chain of reactions leading to the complete metabolic transformation of alcohol takes place in the liver. This

organ in certain individuals may be relatively sensitive to
alcohol, but the latter is no longer considered the sole etiologic agent in cirrhosis of the liver. The normal kidney,
under the influence of moderate amounts of alcohol, is provoked to a variable but minor increase in the quantity of
urine excreted.

It has been demonstrated in animals that alcohol enters
the mother's milk in minute quantities.[13] In human beings,
small amounts of ingested alcohol may be recovered from
the milk of the lactating mother. The amount, in all probability, would be less in the milk of women who are accustomed to alcohol than in the milk of those who are not,
because alcohol is more readily metabolized in those who
are habituated to its use.

The influence of alcohol upon the psyche is recognized
and accepted. Depending upon the tolerance of the person
and the amount consumed, the effect may vary from mild
euphoria to frank anatomic changes in the tissues of the
central nervous system. The reflex mechanisms, particularly
the voluntary or conditioned reflexes, appear to be the most
vulnerable to the effects of alcohol—the more complex the
reflex, the more susceptible it may be.

In regard to the physiologic effects of alcohols other than
ethyl alcohol, which appear in trace quantities in wine, the
following may be recapitulated. The reaction of the human
body to methyl alcohol is quite different from that to ethyl
alcohol. Alterations in intracellular metabolism occur early
and are due to the highly toxic effects of the reduction and
oxidation products of methyl alcohol, formaldehyde, and
formic acid, respectively. In contrast, ethyl alcohol is
promptly transformed into acetaldehyde and finally to carbon dioxide and water. The toxic effect of methyl alcohol is
cumulative because it circulates unchanged within the body
for a relatively long period of time.

The higher alcohols found only in trace quantities are
also toxic, excepting glycerine (glycerol). The amount of

glycerine in wine varies from 3.5 to 13.2 grams per liter. Because of its dilution, its hygroscopic and antiseptic properties are relatively inconsequential. On the other hand, the taste of glycerine is important, particularly for the diabetic. The natural content of glycerine sweetens wines which contain no fermentable sugars, and these are saporifically more agreeable than the saccharine ordinarily prescribed in the diabetic diet. As a matter of fact, no well-fermented natural wine contains more than a trace of fermentable sugars, and for this reason they may be used to brighten any diet restricted in carbohydrate.

From the standpoint of physiologic effects, the organic acids of wine exert characteristic responses. They are found in the free form as well as combined with alcohols, ethereal oils and other aromatic substances. Their effect upon aroma and taste greatly increases the esthetic and physiologic values of wine.[14] In this respect temperature is an important factor because wines have a sharper taste if they are warmed even slightly. Red wines, whose content of organic acids is relatively low, should be served at room temperature and, in general, white wines at about 12° C. In regard to the irritating effects of organic acids, tests on animals, confirmed by human subjective experience, have indicated that lactic and glycolic acids in equimolar solution are the least irritating, followed by tartaric, citric and acetic acids respectively. Because of its ideally balanced proportions, wine is preeminent among all the carriers of organic acid nutrients. Its pH value, which averages 3.2, resembles gastric juice more closely than that of any other natural beverage. In the stomach, the organic acids as present in wine enhance the activity of the pepsin precursors, and in this respect they are as important as the presence of hydrochloric acid in physiologic amounts. In the duodenum, lactic acid reflexly affects the pyloric musculature and suppresses the flow of hydrochloric acid in the gastric juice. On the other hand, acetic acid in the duodenum stimulates the gastric mucous membrane and reflexly provokes the secretion of hydrochloric acid. It is probable that these considerations influence the physiologic effects of certain wines on gastric secretion.

The antiseptic properties of wine are in part due to its content of organic acids, particularly lactic acid which in weak concentration has been shown to inhibit the propagation of certain microorganisms. In a 1 per cent aqueous solution, for instance, lactic acid proves lethal for *S. hemolyticus, S. viridans, N. mucosus capsulatus, Staphylococcus albus,* and *E. coli.* According to Kitasato, quoted by Reich, *E. typhosus* can be killed within four to five hours in the following solutions: 0.4 per cent lactic acid, 0.48 per cent tartaric, citric or malic acids, and 0.28 per cent sulfurous acid. Although it took more than six hours to kill *E. typhosus* when the acids of the wine were neutralized, it died in natural wine within fifteen minutes. In comparing the effects of wine with water containing the same amount of alcohol, it has been demonstrated that the bactericidal action of wine is three times greater than that of water containing a similar concentration of alcohol. Recent investigations have demonstrated that wine possesses antibacterial activity beyond that which can be ascribed to its content of acids, alcohol, tannin or phenols.[15]

The utilization of organic acid is a factor in various metabolic processes. A large part is either burned or transformed into body protein, and the remainder, proportionately small, appears unaltered in the urine as waste products. Lactic, acetic and probably succinic acids are apparently completely decomposed or utilized and leave no detectable residues. Observations on ruminants show that lactic acid is utilized in the intermediary metabolism of carbohydrate and in the synthesis of glycogen in the liver. In this instance the major part of the carbohydrate is transformed into lactic acid in the digestive tract from whence it is reabsorbed, combined with potassium or sodium. In general, the small amounts of organic acids which may enter the circulation unaltered are immediately bound, probably to ammonia, and ultimately burned to supply the body with alkali.

Little is known about the physiologic effects of the esters in wine except that they stimulate the respiratory center. In general, the esters of volatile acids stimulate the olfactory apparatus and are responsible predominantly for the aroma of wine, while the esters of the nonvolatile acids stimulate the gustatory apparatus and are responsible predominantly for the taste of wine.

Carbonic acid occupies a special position among the acids of wine. Being a weak acid with amphoteric qualities, it may exist in the wine as a carbonate or, in varying quantities, as free carbonic acid. In the form of the latter, its effects are localized within the digestive tract where, depending upon the character of the gastric secretions, it is either released as carbon dioxide or it enhances absorption, especially of alcohol. Carbonic acid is odorless, but because it can separate from the wine in the form of fine bubbles it assists in volatilizing the aromatic substances of the wine. In solution, it brings to beverages sharpness and a refreshing taste. It produces a clean effect upon the oral and pharyngeal mucous membrances and alerts the gustatory papillae to new thresholds of stimulation. Carbon dioxide has a local anesthetizing effect, especially in the stomach, and because of this property it has been used therapeutically for the suppression of nausea. Carbonic acid promotes a moderate secretion of hydrochloric acid. Because carbonic acid increases the resorptive capacity of the gastric mucous membrane, the sparkling wines surfeited with carbon dioxide produce euphoria much more rapidly than the noncarbonated wines. Sparkling wines promote diuresis more readily than still wines and in addition, the wines containing carbonic acid may stimulate the heart quickly because of the more prompt absorption of the alcohol they contain.

Tannins produce a puckering effect upon the buccal mucous membrances because they are astringents and precipitate albumin. The tissue-thickening effects they exert upon the mucosae of the stomach and upper gastroenteric tract delay absorption and secretion, and retard motility. In the intestines the tannins combine with alkalis to form tannates; and since these compounds are bound to albumin, their physicochemical reactivity is decreased. Further decomposition of the free tannins liberates gallic acid which exerts only weak astringent powers. Compounds of tannic acid with albumin, insoluble or barely soluble in water, are useful because they separate in the intestine and liberate tannin. The fate of absorbed tannin, tannates, tannin-albuminate and gallic acid is unknown, since only traces of tannic acid can be found in the urine.

Sulfur may appear in wine in its free form as sulfite or bound to acetaldehyde, glucose or fructose. In none of these combinations is it injurious to the human organism. Large amounts of sulfur may impair the aroma and flavor of wine, but, in general, discreet amounts of sulfur enhance the olfactory and gustatory qualities especially of white wines. Often the flower of an elegant white wine is pleasantly perceptible by virtue of the fruity aroma of aldehyde sulfurous acids. In heavily sulfured wines the ill effects are due not so much to the content of sulfur as to the products of faulty fermentation which have been masked by the quantity of sulfur used. Any sulfate which may appear in natural wine would exist as the potassium or sodium salt and it would exert at most a minor laxative effect.

The amount of nitrogenous compounds found in wine is too insignificant to warrant physiologic study. This applies also to the content in wine of boric acid, salicylic acid-ester, silicic acid anhydride and benzoic acid. The mineral, sodium, which appears in natural wine in small quantities, can also be disregarded from the standpoint of its physiologic effects. No definitive statements can be made at this time concerning the physiologic effects of the other mineral elements found in wine. The subject of the trace elements, for instance, is even more highly controversial, as are also the physiologic effects of calcium, the influence of the silicates upon arteriosclerosis and the role of magnesium in phagocytosis. All that can be stated with assurance is that wine contains mineral substances in various quantities conveniently combined in favorable solutions and mixtures.

Tartaric acid exists in wine in the form of potassium tartrate, and as such it exerts a feeble physiologic effect. Only in the presence of alkaline carbonates, as may be found in the intestine, does potassium bitartrate become transformed in part into a neutral salt which then may exert a tartrate effect. Rarely would this amount have any diuretic effect. Certain wines, high in acid and rich in potassium, may produce a distinct polyuria; others, containing the same amount of potassium but with a lower acid content, do not produce this effect even when they contain more alcohol. Therefore, as far as polyuria is concerned, there seems to be a causal relationship between polyuria and the content of acid potassium salt in the wine.

Wines, especially those made from grapes grown in volcanic soil, have been recommended for the feeble and anemic because of their richness in iron and phosphorus. Although the iron requirement of the body varies from 1.0 to 30.0 milligrams per day (average 15 milligrams), the depleted individual because of his specific needs demands more than the normal amount of iron. Some physiologists state that iron-rich wine alone can supply all of the iron necessary for metabolic needs.

Little is known about the physiologic effects of the pigmentary substances of wine, nor has the efficacy of wine as a vehicle for vitamins ever been precisely ascertained. The most difficult objective information to obtain concerns the physiologic effects of the aromatic and taste substances of wine. Until this information becomes exact their physiologic and pharmacologic value cannot be fixed, yet there is no doubt that these substances are responsible for the distinctive character of wine. It is known that some wines, rich in bouquet, influence the heart and circulation; and that others, even in small amounts, may influence the control of the locomotor apparatus. In general, red wines have a more potent, rapid and exciting effect than white wines. This is attributed in part to their content of ethyl acetate and similar compounds. There is no question that wine is the only beverage whose simple origin is by nature destined for the fulfilment of certain human psychologic and physiologic purposes. The grape contains everything necessary to render the final product perfect without the withering touch of man. Wine, next to milk the most complex biologic fluid outside of a blood vessel, with all of its manifold properties resists complete analysis as does the enigma of life.

III. *Wine as Food*

||||||||||||||||||||||||||||||||||||||||||||||||||||||||||||||||||||||||||||||||||||||||||||||||||||||||||||||||||||||||||||||||||||||||||||||||||||||

From the time of Hesiod in the eighth century B.C. wine has been considered an aliment, and as such it plays an important role in the function of nutrition.[1] In pre-Christian Greece, the frugal diet of the Spartan included wine as well as barley meal, cheese, figs, flesh and fish. In Biblical times wine, corn and oil were looked upon as the chief dietary necessities of life, while in the Latin countries, wine goes along with bread among the staples of the national diet.

An aliment is defined as a substance which supplies a factor vitally essential to life or one in which the oxidation in the organism furnishes necessary energy for the exercise of normal physiologic function.[2] Maria Rosa[3] points out that since it has been proved alcohol is an aliment, therefore "wine should be considered an aliment. As such, it merits physiological study just as any other food or medicine does."

Llagnet[4] notes that the French "physicians are truly convinced of the beneficial action of natural wines and their rational use in alimentation." After bread comes wine—the second legacy of the Creator.[5] Empirically all lovers and users of wine, especially those in an advisory capacity such as physicians, consider it a nutritive product of unquestionable value. Among the ancients who praised wine were Hippocrates,[6] Athenaeus,[7] Galens,[8] and Celsus;[9] among the moderns are Guyot,[10] Stoll,[11] Loeper,[12] Lozano,[13] Bunker,[14]

Tant[15] and innumerable others. Dontas[16] says this most tasteful of beverages is at the same time a precious aliment. Its moderate use is salutary. It introduces into the organism many essential and useful alimentary substances: organic and inorganic acids, salts, vitamins, and carbohydrates which act favorably to supply necessary elements for growth, maintenance and repair, as well as fluid and food for energy. According to Jager[17] wine is a precious, economic and common article of the diet which stimulates the gastric secretion without hindering the action of pepsin.

The thirteenth edition of the Encyclopaedia Britannica[18] reports that "so highly did the French military authorities rate wine as a food and medicine during the [first World] War that a full liter became part of every poilu's ration." The purpose of the authorities was to remedy the carbohydrate deficiency in the army diet.[19] In recent times, the Spanish government officially recognized the nutritive value of wine by making it a part of the meal and apportioning its cost on the same basis as bread.[20]

However, it is to be noted that wine contains two types of food elements: those providing energy and those contributing to the maintenance of the body and its nutrition.[21] The nutritive energy element is derived largely from the alcohol which Duhamel[22] has described as the necessary substratum without which wine would not be wine. This is balanced by the vital or maintenance elements. These are the minerals and vitamins present in grapes in varying proportion depending upon the soil in which they are grown and the amount of sunshine and rain which they receive.

In addition to the alcohol, other sources of calories in wine are the simple sugars which are stored as glycogen and converted into glucose when the body requires more energy. Modern wines, depending upon type, may contain from 0.25 to 10 per cent of simple sugars, principally levulose and dextrose—the former with a relative sweetness two-and-one-half times the latter.[23] The role of levulose as a material for maintenance and repair of the liver and as an intermediary substance in metabolism has been demonstrated experimentally by Gettler.[24] Parisi, Sacchetti and Bruini[25] report that in concentrated musts of white grapes subject to the fermentative action of *Zygosaccharomyces*, fructose is attacked preferentially so that its content decreases relative to dextrose. The predominant sugar in these finished wines is dextrose. The dextrose-levulose ratio is used by producers of wine to gauge the completeness of fermentation under controlled conditions for the types of yeasts employed.[26] Most strains of wine yeasts will ferment dextrose faster than levulose; however, the "sauternes yeast" exerts a preferential effect on levulose. It has been shown that physical factors such as the concentration of sugar and the temperature of the fermenting mass may also condition which sugar will be preferentially attacked. As an example, a "sauternes type" of yeast acting in a medium containing less than 20 per cent total sugar will show a preferential fermentation of dextrose; between 20 and 25 per cent sugar, both dextrose and levulose will be fermented at nearly equal rates; beyond 25 per cent total sugar, the preference will be for the selective fermentation of levulose. Such behavior of a given strain of yeast is postulated as the resultant of its action upon the original concentration of sugar, its affinity for the enzyme, hexokinase, and its rate of penetration through cell walls.[27] Every physician recognizes that the rapid absorption and complete availability of dextrose (d-glucose) makes it an immediately useful energy food. In addition it is also a protective agent for all tissues of the body. The speed of absorption of dextrose is particularly important when metabolic requirements are excessive.[28] Connor[29] and Chaikoff[30] consider dextrose the most important single factor in the prevention of fatty infiltration of the liver, a condition which they believe predisposes this organ to cirrhosis.

Two further points are to be considered in the discussion of wine as a source of energy:

(*1*) Alcohol does not impede the absorption of dextrose, a fact which was early demonstrated by Tappeiner,[31] Brandl,[32] and von Scanzoni,[33] and more recently confirmed by the researches of Higgins,[34] Edkins,[35] and Murray working with Edkins.[36]

(*2*) At least 95 per cent of the energy of alcohol is readily available for immediate use. This value was first established by Neumann,[37] whose work was subsequently substantiated by Atwater and Benedict.[38] These conclusions refute the prejudicial statement that alcohol is not burned by the organism.

The low nitrogen content of wine precludes its classification among protein foods. "Nevertheless," Dougnac[39] states, "it contains a certain proportion of proteids in the form of amino acids [which are] directly assimilable." In children, a significant rise in hemoglobin following the daily ingestion of grape juice was recorded by Fishbein, Calvin and Heumann.[40] This effect may be attributed to the amino acids, iron or vitamins embodied in this nutrient substance. Wine also contains other organic materials of nutritional value such as purines, pectins, fats, inulin and glyccrine. Although the quantities of these substances are small, each has a recognized value as a food and potential therapeutic agent.

The essential nutritional constituents of wine vary with the conditions under which the grape grows and matures. Wine has been found by Randoin,[41] Morgan and co-workers,[42] and others to contain consistent and measurable quantities of the B vitamins in sufficient amounts to add substantially to the daily vitamin intake.

As for minerals, modern wines contain, in some degree, all thirteen of the elements Underwood[43] considers necessary for the maintenance of animal and human life: calcium, phosphorus, magnesium, sodium, potassium, chlorine, sulfur, iron, copper, manganese, zinc, iodine, and cobalt. A list of the mineral constituents of wine musts indicates that they contain favorable and utilizable amounts of the more important minerals potassium, magnesium, sodium, calcium, iron and phosphorus.[44] The content of sodium in the ash of natural wine fluctuates between 10 and 60 or more milligrams per liter. Under modern conditions of production, vinification, and stabilization of the wines, the sodium content may vary from 26 to 400 milligrams per liter, with an average figure of 85 milligrams per liter. The higher values are in all probability due to the addition of sodium-containing compounds to the wine in the course of its production.[45] The question of the sodium content of wines is of importance to patients on a sodium-restricted diet, and for that reason selected samples of some California table wines* were subjected to analysis for sodium and potassium content. For the sodium analysis the wine was ashed and then diluted 1:2; for the potassium analysis the wine was diluted 1:50; the values for both were determined on a Perkin-Elmer Flame Photometer. The tests were all done in duplicate. The sodium and potassium values were as follows:

	Sodium milligrams per liter	Potassium milligrams per liter
Mountain Zinfandel 1945	25.8	1053.0
Mountain Folle Blanche	14.7	624.0
Napa Burgundy	68.0	1055.7
Barbera	51.1	958.0
Mountain Sylvaner	25.8	645.1
Mountain Zinfandel 1947	12.9	762.5
Cabernet Sauvignon	13.3	1055.0
Napa Chianti	25.3	977.5
California Dry Sauterne	39.1	899.3

The contents of potassium, phosphate and copper regularly found in wine are of individual significance in main-

---

* These wines were made available by L. M. Martini of St. Helena, California.

taining, respectively, the rhythmicity of the normal heart beat, the metabolic equilibrium in the utilization of dextrose,[46] and the synthesis and regeneration of hemoglobin.[47] In addition, aluminum, manganese and other elements are also present in trace quantities.

The study of Saywell and Cunningham[48] established the facts that 80 per cent of the iron present in wine is in the reduced or ferrous form—easily absorbed from the intestinal tract—and also that the reduced iron in wine is stable and utilizable after long periods of aging. They further noted that the moderate use of wine at mealtime supplies adults with an adequate daily iron supplement, an important factor in the iron-deficient diet of the average American.

Finally, there are other substances in wine—such as aromatic esters, some of which defy exact chemical analysis and whose physiologic activity as yet remains unknown, but whose presence contributes to the pleasant aroma and bouquet of the beverage and ensures palatability to many diets—all of which make wine the beverage that we know.

Experimentally it has been demonstrated that wine in certain proportions acts as a substitute for energy food and as a promoter of protein storage. If the amount of wine is not excessive, it can replace in the diet isodynamic quantities of fats and carbohydrates.[49] An American commission called "The Committee of Fifty" established similar conclusions in regard to alcohol after carefully conducted experimentation in which an attempt was made to shed light upon the nutritive value of alcohol when taken in moderate quantities. Many of the experiments were performed by Atwater and his associates.[50] One such experiment involved three healthy subjects—an American, a Swede, and a Canadian—who ranged in age from twenty-five to thirty-three. During the experiment their weights remained constant. One had always used fermented beverages in moderation and the other two were teetotalers. Each was placed in a calorimetric chamber where he was free to move about and do as he was directed. The heat production of their bodies was measured accurately. The food they ingested was calculated in order to establish scientifically the metabolic factors of the ingested substances, and all of their excretions were analyzed quantitatively. Seventy-two grams of absolute alcohol divided in six portions (three taken with the meals, three between meals) were provided as a daily supplement to the dietary ration. The alcohol supplied 20 per cent of the total calories in the "rest experiment" and 14 per cent in the "work experiment."

The experiment showed that alcohol in the quantities ingested has a physiologic action as useful as the principal foods for which it was substituted. It replaces protein, fat and carbohydrate isodynamically. Within certain limits, it can replace fats, carbohydrates and proteins as a producer of heat. Alcohol acts as a food which protects protein as well as other tissue substances when it is utilized as a source of heat or for energy purposes.[51]

Albertoni and Rossi[52] reached similar conclusions with experiments upon peasants who were accustomed to a strictly vegetable diet and who did not use wine. A balanced diet was given to the subjects and careful analyses of aliquots of the food, feces and urine were done. During the test period of twenty days they added one-half liter of wine to the daily food ration and repeated the analyses. These authors concluded that (1) as the amount of food in the basic ration diminished while the subjects were taking wine, the caloric value of the total daily allowance of food was elevated and the calories generated by the metabolized alcohol were utilized directly in the maintenance of body temperature, and indirectly in producing energy; (2) the nitrogen balance, which was negative during the preliminary period of the trial diet, became definitely positive following the ingestion of wine, an evidence of the protein-sparing effect of wine.

Richter[53] has shown that rats, when allowed to incorporate in their diet dilute solutions (1 to 6 per cent) of alcohol in place of water, selected alcohol among the group of substances having nutritional value. The dilute solutions of alcohol were incorporated in the diet without disturbing its total caloric content. When forced to take larger amounts of alcohol, the rats reduced their food intake in almost direct proportion to the increase in the calories obtained from the alcohol. Since they grew and apparently thrived under these circumstances, it is concluded that alcohol may replace certain amounts of food in the diet. Of primary importance is the fact that the total caloric intake, regardless of the amount of alcohol ingested, was not increased beyond its normal level.

From these experiments it is not to be implied that wine can replace all other foods. Rather it should be considered in the daily ration as a source of calories, as a stomachic and as an important adjuvant.[54] Cuvier[55] is of the opinion that "wine should be drunk with meals, rarely between meals and always in proportions suitable to the organism." Some recommend that it be consumed in the same quantities as other nutritive substances.[56] On the other hand, Clauera[57] maintains that metabolically the normal organism can handle as a daily maximum about 1 gram of alcohol per kilogram of body weight; this corresponds, in general, to about 800 to 1,000 cubic centimeters of wine. For women this would be reduced by approximately one-third. Each individual reacts differently depending upon his state of health and his tolerance. According to Weissenbach,[58] some of the factors to be considered in the consumption of wine as a food are "age, sex, profession, constitution, race, customs, ancestral habits, climate and surroundings."

Wine can be recommended without qualification for persons who derive great benefit from living out of doors, especially sportsmen. For them wine is a source of strength and vigor and an addition to the joy of an unrestricted appetite. For the sedentary, the idle, the infirm and the convalescent it is a valuable nutriment when taken in proportion.

Since he who drinks wine requires less carbohydrate than ordinarily, alcohol obviously is a factor to be considered in the treatment of obesity. It is never to be prohibited arbitrarily without understanding the part it might play in the psychologic conditioning of the person. In the treatment of obesity, wine can be used, but it must be prescribed with precision and great art. Jager[59] points out that the use of wine varies with the cause of the obesity. In the endogenous type, white wine is preferred because of its diuretic properties and its stimulating effect on neuromuscular tone. In exogenous obesity, the caloric content of the wine consumed should not exceed the number of calories which would be obtained from the carbohydrate it replaces. Christie[60] adds the following admonitions:

(*1*) The merely plump should avoid rich, heavy wines as sedulously as they do the solids. (A glass of Burgundy is equivalent to three lumps of sugar, champagne to four-and-one-half.)

(*2*) The daily quota of alcohol for the definitely obese should be stated clearly in the dietetic prescription and apportioned in terms of glasses. The caloric value must be deducted from the total dietary allowance.

(*3*) An absolute maximum of 16 per cent of the energy value of a low caloric, slow-reducing diet may be allotted to alcohol without disturbing the proper balance between essential foods. The best alcohol value for a low calorie diet is to be obtained by choosing table wines comparatively free from carbohydrates. Furthermore, the amount of wine allotted must never be exceeded. The converse of the above would, of course, be prescribed in the treatment of the thin and undernourished person.

In order to enjoy the salutary effect of wine to the utmost, it should be included in the diet regularly and in proportion

TABLE OF AVERAGE CALORIC VALUES OF SOME CALIFORNIA WINES*

Type	Calories from Alcohol	Calories from Extract	Calories per 100 cc.	Calories per ounce**
Table Wines, Red				
Barbera	87.5	11.6	99	29
Burgundy	86.1	11.6	98	29
Burgundy, sparkling	81.9	18.8	101	30
Cabernet	89.6	11.6	101	30
Champagne, pink	81.2	16.4	98	29
Chianti	88.9	11.2	100	30
Claret	84.7	12.4	97	29
Zinfandel	88.9	11.2	100	30
Table Wines, White				
Chablis	81.2	9.2	90	27
Champagne	87.5	13.2	101	30
Hock, Moselle, Rhine	85.4	8.8	94	28
Riesling	82.6	9.2	92	27
Sauterne	84.0	10.4	94	28
Sauterne, dry	82.6	9.2	92	27
Sauterne, sweet	86.1	18.4	104	31
Sweet Wines				
Angelica	135.1	52.8	188	55
Aromatic wine (vermouth type)	113.4	75.2	189	56
Muscat	135.8	54.0	190	56
Madeira	135.1	36.4	172	51
Marsala	135.1	38.0	173	51
Port, White	137.2	50.8	188	55
Sherry	139.3	22.0	161	47
Sherry (dry)	138.6	18.8	157	46
Sweet Red Wine	137.2	50.4	188	55
Tokay	134.4	46.4	181	53

* The caloric values of wines are expressed as average numbers of calories of many samples of wines of each type. The values were derived by multiplying the average alcoholic content in grams per 100 cubic centimeters by 7 calories per gram; and the average content of extracts expressed in grams per 100 cubic centimeters times 4 calories per gram. The ultimate figure grossly approximates the value of 7 calories per gram of alcohol, 4.1 calories per gram of carbohydrates and 4.3 calories per gram of glycerine.

** For purposes of this calculation, the figure of 29.6 cubic centimeters per ounce was used and the caloric value estimated to the nearest round figure.

to any other healthful food rather than taken sporadically. The argument that in moderate amounts wine or alcohol poisons the organism is as groundless as the statement that meat or sugar endangers the lives of those who eat them. All three are foods, and indeed important in the normal and well-rounded life. Good wine in the diet is one of the most stimulating aliments in the nutrition of man. These statements are "supported by research on various groups of human beings whatever their degree of civilization."[61]

It can be stated, then, that wine is an aliment containing two types of food elements: those providing energy and those contributing to the maintenance of the body and its nutrition. The energy element is derived chiefly from the carbohydrates, including alcohol; the vital maintenance elements are derived from the minerals, vitamins, and other constituents of wine. In addition to its caloric value, the moderate daily use of wine contributes four important elements to the well-balanced diet:

(*1*) Natural hexoses (dextrose and levulose), the predominant sugars in finished wine, which are easily absorbed and assimilated.

(*2*) The vitamin B complex in sufficient quantity to augment substantially the daily intake of these necessary factors. (Wine is the only alcoholic beverage commonly used which contains proven quantities of physiologically active B complex vitamins).

(*3*) An adequate supplement of iron in active form which can be absorbed easily from the intestine.

(*4*) Many mineral elements necessary to health.

Wine has proved itself to be a valuable adjunct to the daily diet of the human subject regardless of his economic status or social position. It serves as an agent to alter physiologic functions which can be measured and to influence psychologic states which can be conditioned.

IV. *The Action of Wine upon the Digestive Organs and Its Use in Diseases of the Gastrointestinal System*

‖‖‖

In 1595, in his "Government of Health," Dr. William Bullein[1] wrote, "They that drinke wyne customably with measure, it doth profit them much and maketh good digestion; those people that use to drinke wyne seldom times, be distempered."

Since Dr. Bullein's day, clinicians have ascertained that wine not only maintains the harmony of the digestive function in general, but that it also affects each organ individually. The extent of this effect is determined by three factors: (*1*) the character and strength of the wine; (*2*) the amount; and (*3*) the frequency of the quantity ingested. It is to be noted that the primary function of wine in the digestive process is as a stimulant of the appetite. In the cocktail, ordinarily considered an apéritif, the content of alcohol is so great that its physiologic effects as a depressant predominate. Wine, on the other hand, through its lower content of alcohol, its ethers, aroma and flavor, excites the olfactory sense, the gustatory papillae and the digestive functions.[2] In addition, Trullols[3] comments on its therapeutic value as a stimulator of the appetite. Mallory[4] is of the opinion that when taken for such a purpose wine does not contain a sufficient quantity of alcohol to contraindicate its use.

Closely allied to the function of wine as an apéritif is the psychic effect by which the whole digestive process is set in motion. According to Pachon,[5] the automatic release by reflex action of the gastric secretions is the "principal and primordial action" of wine. In reference to this "veritable psychic secretion," Loeper and Alquier[6] believe that the taste and even the bouquet of wine influence the reaction.

The quantity of wine ingested influences the character of the digestive responses. Port or sherry, in portions of a wine glass or so, act purely as stimulants. In larger amounts they appreciably retard digestion. Oddly enough, this inhibitory action, Billings[7] found, bears no relationship to the content of alcohol, but rather to the residues or solid matters of wine. The results of his research are in accord with those of Sir William Roberts[8] who showed that in a mixture containing 40 per cent of port or sherry, the action of the digestive processes was retarded. Even though such an amount of wine is equivalent to only 20 per cent of absolute alcohol (which has been shown to have little effect on digestion), sherry prolonged the time required to complete digestion. From this research, Roberts and his colleagues concluded that the retarding action of wine must be due to some agent other than alcohol. Experiments repeated with light French and stronger Hungarian wines[9] produced similar though less marked results; the retarding effect proved to be independent of the concentration of alcohol present.

Billings[10] cites experimental data to substantiate his viewpoint that the retarding action is due to various factors of unknown nature which make up the solid matters in wine (in a sample of sherry which he used this amounted to 4.75 per cent). "Further, it is evident that this solid matter, when free from the alcohol of the wine, has by itself a distinct influence on peptic digestion." Billings summarized these effects as follows: (*1*) a definite retardation of digestion attributed to the solid residues obtained from the sherry, and (*2*) a weaker stimulatory effect, *i.e.,* increasing the rate of digestion, which he attributed to the volatile substances of the sherry, namely alcohol, ethers and aromatic substances. The increase in the rate of digestion due to the volatile substances may be nullified by the content or nature of the solid residues in wine or possibly by the alcohol itself free from a higher proportion of volatile substances other than alcohol. "Obviously, however, if sherry be mixed with gastric juice in such quantity as to introduce five, ten or fifteen per cent of absolute alcohol, the latter will produce its ordinary retardation of proteolytic action, although doubtless lessened somewhat by the bouquet or other volatile material which apparently stimulates rather than retards peptic digestion."

White wines are less active than red wines in delaying pepsin-proteolysis. This, according to Billings,[11] stems from the fact that as a rule they contain less solid matters than red. Carlson[12] reaches a similar conclusion and states that "sour wines cause greater inhibition than the sweet wines— probably through their acids."

In concluding the discussion of the effects of alcohol upon the stomach and digestive processes, it may be said that (*1*) wine in small quantities, such as would be included in the normal diet, exerts a stimulating action; (*2*) taken in larger amounts, wine tends to impede the chemical processes of digestion by virtue of the depressant effect of alcohol and/or its content of solid residues.

Effects on the Salivary Glands

Roberts[13] maintains that wine inhibits salivary secretion, although his predecessor, Beaurepaire[14] stated that wine causes the glands to secrete saliva more abundantly. Experiments by the modern authorities, Loeper and Alquier[15] corroborate the findings of Beaurepaire. They state that if one retains in the mouth a spoonful of wine and some food, the quantity of ptyalin in the salivary secretion is increased. This may be attributed to a direct effect of wine on salivary secretion and a secondary effect leading to the increased digestion of starches. Chittenden and associates[16] previously had found that the application of strong concentrations of alcohol to the tongue excited the salivary flow, whereas the introduction of alcohol directly into the stomach did not. During a detailed investigation, Winsor and Strongin[17] observed that the salivary flow increased for a ten-minute period following the ingestion of moderate amounts of wine and that after one and one-half hours, the rate of secretion returned to a basal level. The cause of the increase in salivary flow is not definitely known. Beazell and Ivy[18] have offered the most satisfactory opinion to date, namely, that the increased flow is due to direct sensitization of the secretory nerve endings in the salivary glands.

It has been demonstrated experimentally that the concentration of alcohol in the saliva parallels that in the arterial blood due, in all probability, to diffusion. These relationships have been studied by Linde,[19] Abels,[20] Vollenbruck,[21] and Friedmann and co-workers.[22] As a result of these researches, the salivary excretion levels are now accepted in medicolegal work.

Effect on the Tongue and the Esophagus

As noted above, wine excites the papillae of the tongue. Ordinarily there is no absorption from the esophagus because of the rapidity with which wine passes through the esophagus and the unfitness of the mucosa for absorption. However, absorption can take place in the esophagus if previously it has been irritated or damaged by the passage through it of concentrated solutions of alcohol[23] or if the mechanism of its emptying is interfered with.

Effects on the Stomach

As has been noted above, dilute concentrations of alcohol increase the motility of the stomach.[24] Strong concentrations, on the other hand, have a definite delaying action. This conclusion is borne out by Carlson,[25] who found that hunger contractions were inhibited for one to two hours after the ingestion of 10 per cent solutions of alcohol. Saito[26] was among the first of the physiologists to show that alcohol in concentrations of 7 to 20 per cent augments the gastric flow. The observation has been verified by Babkin,[27] Barlow,[28] and Dragstedt and associates.[29] The latter suggest that the alcohol stimulates gastric secretion by a primary liberation of histamine. The secretogogue effect of alcohol is of practical importance since it has been used in various tests of gastric secretion. The studies of Barlow[30] reveal that concentrations of alcohol above 20 per cent definitely irritate the gastric mucosa. This provokes a defensive outpouring of mucus which is secreted as a protection against the toxic effects of such concentrations of alcohol. The mechanics of the effects of wine on the gastric mucosa have not as yet precisely been determined. Nevertheless it may be assumed that the gastric secretion is augmented in one or more of the following ways:

(*a*) Direct nonirritative contact with the gastric mucosa.

(*b*) Direct action on the secreting cells through diffusion from the blood stream.

(*c*) Reflex stimulation through the vagus nerve. The sensory pathway is assumed to be mediated through the afferent nerves of the mouth, pharynx and stomach.

(*d*) Relaxation of mental tension which thereby releases cerebral inhibitions.

According to Mareschalchi,[31] wine exhibits a stimulant effect on the smooth muscle of the stomach. It provokes energetic peristaltic movement and at the same time produces maximal effects on the digestive function and emptying time of the stomach. In temperate amounts, the alcoholic content of table wine activates the stomach, accelerates gastric secretion and brings forth from the secreting mucosa a gastric juice rich in sodium chloride, hydrochloric acid and the enzymes rennin and pepsin.[32]

The increase in the flow of pepsin after the ingestion of alcohol was observed by Kast[33] and by Lönnquist,[34] early in the nineteenth century. Babkin,[35] as well as Krueger and MacIntosh,[36] confirmed these observations. The increase in the quantity of pepsin is not of the same order as the increase of hydrochloric acid. However, due to the augmented flow of gastric secretion, there is an absolute increase in the total pepsin produced. Persons suffering from inadequate gastric digestion following the usual mixed meal will be interested in the study made by Haneborg[37] who showed that the ingestion of diluted alcohol with mixed meals increases the proteolytic power of the gastric juice. It should be remembered that the secretory augmentation which follows the ingestion of wine differs from that following the ingestion of plain solutions of alcohol. Ogden[38] has demonstrated that the sustained stimulation of gastric secretion characteristic of wine is independent of its content of alcohol although the amount of secretion within certain limits is dependent upon the concentration of alcohol. In wine, the natural fruit salts, tartrates, phosphates and other constituents act as buffers to check the high concentration of acids characteristic of unbuffered solutions. The buffering effect causes a tempered increase in the flow of gastric juice which extends over a longer period of time and which is more in harmony with the natural digestive and propulsive factors of gastric digestion.

In order to determine the effect of an amount of wine comparable to a pre-dinner appetizer, Scott and his co-workers[39] gave a glassful of 20 per cent alcohol (the usual concentration in dessert or appetizer wine) followed in five minutes by a second glassful with the same alcoholic content. After a lapse of five minutes, they observed definite hunger sensations and noted a relaxation of gastric tension which accompanied the increased hunger contractions for almost an hour. In view of the present-day stress of living, such a preprandial effect should be an important factor in the prevention of the all-too-prevalent dyspepsias.

Effect on the Intestines

The difficulties of an experimental approach to digestion in the small intestine are such that few references are available; nor are there a great many more on the effects of wine in the large intestine. However, as long ago as 1831 Beaurepaire[40] pronounced the effects of wine on the intestine as both good and desirable. One of the factors most highly recommended is the antiseptic action wine exercises upon the content of the intestinal tract.[41] Ferrannini attributes the bactericidal power of wine to the amount of aromatic ethers it contains: "that is why old wines have been considered better in this respect, as their ethers are enhanced by age in the bottle."[42]

In recent years, Adler, Beazell, Atkinson and Ivy[43] have observed in human subjects with colostomies that alcohol in 20 per cent concentration increases the propulsive activity of the colon. A similar concentration of alcohol given to normal subjects facilitates the gastrocolic reflex, thereby aiding natural evacuation of the colon.

Effect on the Pancreas

Experiments performed by Kuwschinski[44] before the turn of the century showed that the flow of pancreatic juice was increased after the administration of alcohol. Similar observations have been reported frequently, although the precise mechanism of this action was not critically evaluated. It was also demonstrated that alcohol was an effective pancreatic stimulant whether administered by stomach or by rectum,[45] or even when introduced into a closed intestinal loop.[46] However, the experiments of Brooks and Thomas[47] have demonstrated that dilute alcohol has very little direct stimulating effect upon the volume or the enzymatic activity of the external secretion of the pancreas when instilled directly into the duodenum or given intravenously to dogs equipped with duodenal and gastric fistulas. These experiments indicate that the probable mechanism of action of alcohol on the pancreas consists of primary stimulation of the secretion of hydrochloric acid and secondary stimulation of the pancreas by the gastric juice as it enters the duodenum. In human beings Dreiling[48] found that alcohol has no direct stimulating effect upon the pancreatic secretions collected through a duodenal tube. An increased flow of pancreatic juice is usually accompanied by a proportionate increase in the output of pancreatic enzymes and these are highly important factors in digestion. Because of the stimulatory effect of wine on the pancreas, it should be given with care to patients suffering from any impairment of pancreatic function; furthermore, when used in such instances, its effects should be carefully observed.

Effects on the Liver

Ingested wine is transported to the liver from the intestinal tract by way of the portal vein. Since it is freely diluted with intestinal juices, it reaches the liver in weak concentrations. However, wine is an aliment to which the liver responds more readily[49] and dilution in no way impedes its stimulatory effect on hepatic function.[50] The effect of wine upon the hepatic cell may provoke one or more of the following reactions: (1) increase in the flow of bile into the duodenum; (2) alter the nitrogen coefficient; (3) alter the coefficient of Maillard; (4) produce variations in the coefficient of sulfur oxidation.

In 1929, Loeper, Michaux and de Seze[51] administered wine by duodenal tube and by mouth to two groups of subjects, normal persons and patients with liver disease. In the first experiment, the introduction by duodenal tube of 20 cubic centimeters of wine provoked a flow of 190 cubic centimeters of bile. (Sweet wines and white wines proved to be more stimulating than red table wines.) In the control experiment, the volume of bile secreted following a 20 cubic centimeters duodenal installation of magnesium sulfate was less than 100 cubic centimeters. In the second experiment, the authors gave wine orally to healthy subjects and to young subjects suffering from hepatic disorders. They then determined the variation in the nitrogen coefficient and the coefficient of Maillard. In normal subjects and those affected with minor, or curable, hepatitis, the oral ingestion of wine caused an elevation in the nitrogen coefficient and a diminution of the coefficient of Maillard. The curve of the variations in the coefficient of sulfur paralleled that of the nitrogen utilization. These data demonstrate that in this experiment wine facilitated the assimilation of nitrogen and at the same time stimulated deamination by the liver. However, if the liver is seriously damaged, the nitrogen coefficient is depressed and the coefficient of Maillard is increased, both of which alterations indicate hepatic insufficiency. According to these authors, wine serves a useful purpose in the prognosis of hepatic disorders. An overly-excitable liver reacts to it more readily than a normal liver; a diseased liver does not respond as well. Loeper, Michaux and de Seze use this information clinically as follows: they administer orally 200 cubic centimeters of white wine in the fasting state and examine the urine before and after its ingestion. A calculation of the coefficients tells the story.

There are two misconceptions concerning the effect of alcohol on the liver which should be discussed. One concerns the statement that the regular consumption of wine may produce hepatic lesions in an otherwise healthy liver; the other, that wine can be the determining factor in the production of cirrhosis. These statements are frank exaggerations unsupported by any evidence and are usually made by prejudiced persons. An excess of any aliment or medicament or any substance, beneficial when taken in moderation, may prove toxic and cause hepatic disease if the liver is in unstable physiologic balance due to any number of causes. A vulnerable liver becomes insufficient or cirrhotic due to the misuse and not to the moderate use of these substances. Under normal conditions, wine included discreetly in the diet does not produce hepatic lesions.[52] On the contrary, when taken in moderation, it enhances the functions of the liver. Wine as the causative factor of cirrhosis is exceedingly rare except in those who use it excessively and to the exclusion of any other food substance. Cirrhosis, Valin[53] states, is produced by concentrated alcohol—not the small amount found in wine but the high percentage present in spirituous drinks (provided that dietary insufficiency is co-existent). Mauriac[54] declares: "It is the abuse of alcohol which causes cirrhosis of the liver. It has been demonstrated that wine plays no part in the production of this disease." "Those who have cirrhosis," Fiessinger[55] observes, "are generally the alcoholics . . . moderate drinkers of wine do not have to fear that malady."

Wine is widely used in the treatment of diseases of the digestive system. It is found to be particularly beneficial in anorexia, hypochlorhydria without gastritis and hyposthenic dyspepsia. Minor hepatic insufficiency responds not unfavorably to unadulterated dry white table wine. The tannin content and the mildly antiseptic properties of wine make it valuable in the treatment of intestinal colic, mucous colitis, spastic constipation, diarrhea and many infectious diseases of the gastrointestinal tract. By virtue of the anesthetic effect of carbon dioxide, champagne or effervescent wines give excellent results in prolonged nausea and in vomiting caused by gastric irritation. The diuretic effect of white wines appears to be advantageous in certain disorders of the urogenital system.

Wine is contraindicated in any disease of the digestive system characterized by hyperacidity or where there are indications of potential gastroduodenal hemorrhage. Gastritis, pyloric stenosis, ulcers or cancer of the stomach definitely preclude the use of wine in any form. Because of its stimulating effect on the quantity and rate of flow of the pancreatic secretion, wine is contraindicated in acute inflammation of the pancreas as well as in conditions associated with biliary dysfunction.

In addition to its general therapeutic action on the digestive processes, wine exerts beneficial effects on the individual organs which make up the gastrointestinal tract. In the salivary glands it causes a marked increase in flow due, in all probability, to the stimulation of the secretory nerve endings. Under ordinary circumstances, wine is not absorbed in the esophagus. High concentrations of alcohol, as in spirits, irritate the gastric mucosa, but wine low in alcoholic content is highly beneficial. Wine induces a secretion of gastric juice rich in sodium chloride, hydrochloric acid and in the enzymes rennin and pepsin. Although the literature available on the action of wine in the jejunum, ileum and colon is sparse, indications are that physically it produces therapeutic results. In the pancreas, the action is analogous to that in the salivary glands. Contrary to common opinion, alcohol in moderation seems to have a beneficial and stimulant effect on the liver.

For the guidance of clinicians who find gastric oenotherapy not only permissible but desirable, the following suggestions are offered :[56]

(*1*) Prohibit wine altogether until a specific diagnosis can be made and a logical therapeutic regimen can be instituted.

(*2*) When indicated, prescribe wine wisely and in moderation for both its psychologic and physiologic effects.

(*3*) Tonic wines are best taken on an empty stomach before the principal meals. Beverage and table wines are appropriately given with the dietetic prescription.

(*4*) The amount of wine to be taken should be gauged by the condition of the patient and the character of his illness. From two to four ounces—neat or diluted, according to indications—may be given with considerable profit.

(5) Moderately sweet wines are most highly recommended because they are palatable stimulants of vital functions and offer calories as well as analgetic benefits. Light, aged red wines are beneficial, especially in convalescence. Wines rich in tannin are indicated in disorders of the bowel characterized by hypermotility and/or hypersecretion.

(6) Generally contraindicated are the highly alcoholized wines unless they are diluted. In this fashion they may be used most effectively when fluids are to be forced.

(7) Young or yeasty wines are best avoided.

(8) Wines should be discontinued upon the appearance of symptoms of intolerance.

V. The Action of Wine upon the Respiratory System

In regard to the physiologic effect of beverage alcohol on the lung and respiratory apparatus, Billings[1] quotes the experiments of Krautweg (1893) and Vogel (1897), whose studies of the action of the volatile constituents of alcoholic beverages showed that these constituents are more powerful as respiratory stimulants both in animals and man than is ethyl alcohol. The general statement made by physicians that highly flavored wines are better respiratory stimulants than plain wines is supported by these experiments. Wendelstadt[2] demonstrated that alcoholic beverages such as wines and brandies, which contain large amounts of esters, have an even more pronounced stimulating effect on the respiratory volume than ethyl alcohol. In his experiments, he measured the effects of pure alcohol, of cognac, and of various wines on a number of persons primarily for the purpose of testing the reactions in conditions of bodily weariness. In all the experiments in which pure alcohol was used, sugar and lemon juice were added to render it palatable. His findings are summarized in the tables on pp. 62 and 63.

In regard to the level of alcohol in the blood and in the alveolar capillaries, LeBreton[3] noted that it becomes rapidly equilibrated with that of the systemic circulation. Any volatile substance in the alveolar blood diffuses into the alveolar air in accordance with Henry's law of diffusion of gases (*i.e.,* the concentration in blood is proportional to the partial pressure of the gas in the alveoli, the temperature remaining constant). Southgate and Carter[4] state that 2 liters of expired air contain as much alcohol as 1 cubic centimeter of blood. The conclusions of Harger, Lamb and

Effects on the Respiratory Volume
I. Effect of Ethyl Alcohol

Subject	Ethyl alcohol given in cc.	Percentage gain or loss in the respiration volume
VIII.	5	+0.45
VIII.	15	+1.17
II.	15	+9.09
II.	15	+9.57
I.	15	+9.84
VI.	15	−11.02
VI.	15	−7.75
VII.	20	+6.39
V.	20	+2.89
IV.	20	+8.62
V.	25	+7.29
V.	40	+12.16
V.	60	+4.78

II. Effect of Wines

Subject	Amount of alcohol in the wines given in cc.	Kind of wine	Percentage gain or loss in the respiration volume
II.	4.25	Sherry	+7.70
I.	4.25	"	+9.14
II.	8.50	"	+7.71
I.	8.50	"	+3.09
V.	11.50	Rhine wine	+6.74
II.	12.75	Sherry	+14.61
VIII.	17	"	+9.80
V.	17	"	−7.58
II.	17	"	+9.82
I.	17	"	+7.83
IV.	25	"	+48.34
III.	40	Champagne	+14.14
V.	51	Sherry	+49.24
V.	60	Cognac	+24.01

III. Effect of Ethyl Alcohol and Wine on Persons Exhausted
by Labor or Exercise

Subject	Amount of alcohol given in cc.	Percentage gain or loss in the respiration volume
VIII.	5	+23.11
V.	10	+54.17
VI.	15	+25.75
V.	20	+42.09
IV.	20	+77.09
IV.	20	+50.46
VII.	20	+52.34
V.	60	+92.26
V.	17 in form of sherry	+83.60
V.	18 in form of cognac	+96.82

Wendelstadt has also tabulated the results of his predecessors in forms corresponding to his own as given below.

IV. Effect of Wines on Non-fatigued Persons

Person	Amount of alcohol in cc. in wine given	Kind of wine	Percentage gain or loss in resp. vol.
Weissenfeld H.	7.45	Malt wine	+16.19
" A.	8.5	Sherry	+54.39
" B.	8.5	"	+55.80
" D.	8.5	"	+4.67
" G.	10.25	"	+30.90
" J.	11.0	Malt wine	+14.51
" K.	11.0	" "	+22.58
Willmanns, I.	12.0	Sherry	+16.99
Weissenfeld C.	12.75	"	+61.56
" E.	12.75	"	+24.51
" F.	12.75	"	+70.97
Willmanns II.	22.5	"	+30.60
Geppert I.	25	Port wine	+9.0
" I.	60	Cognac	+6.0
" I.	60	(Rhine Wine) (Mousseux)	+15.7
" I.	75	Cognac	+9.2
Vierordt A.	80	Mosel wine	+0.19
" B.	80	" "	−10.71
Geppert IV.	125	Cognac	−1.3
" IV.	125	"	+26.7
" IV.	190	"	+16.2

Hulpieu[5] corroborate the findings of their British colleagues. In true alveolar air, Haggard and Greenberg[6] found the ratio to be 1 in the blood to 1,142 in the alveolar air. They estimated that as much as 8 per cent of alcohol taken orally might be eliminated via the pulmonary ventilation. The effect of forced increase of ventilation on the rate of alcohol excretion has been studied by several investigators: Hunter and Mudd; Robinson and Selesnick; and McFarland and Barach.[7] A decided clinical improvement manifested by a decrease in the concentration of alcohol in the blood was noted following the inhalation of "stimulating" mixtures of oxygen and carbon dioxide. Although the rate of excretion of alcohol through the respired air increased during the inhalation of carbon dioxide-oxygen mixtures, Newman and Card[8] observed that the total amount of alcohol in the body was not appreciably reduced and that following withdrawal of forced ventilation of the mixture of gases, the concentration of alcohol in the blood returned to its former level.

Following the oral ingestion of concentrated alcoholic beverages, the respiratory rate increases momentarily. This effect is due to stimulation of sensory reflexes in the mouth and pharynx. Wine taken by mouth does not produce any sensory shock so that the temporary increase in pulmonary ventilation characteristic of concentrated alcohol does not take place. Brooks[9] stated that solutions containing 50 per cent to 60 per cent alcohol effect no increase in rate, rhythm or depth of ventilation when administered by stomach tube or gastric fistula or when given intravenously. These findings were confirmed by Hyatt.[10]

In studies of the basal metabolism following the ingestion of 10 per cent alcohol, Grubbs and Hitchcock[11] observed no changes either in the ventilation equivalent or in the alveolar carbon dioxide content. They did not find that the ingestion of alcohol exerted any specific dynamic effect on the basal metabolic rate.

The therapeutic use of wines in the treatment of acute respiratory infections enjoyed great popularity among the ancient Greek and Roman physicians[12] as well as among the physicians of Latin countries in recent centuries. Graham[13] commented upon the use of berry wines and wines made from various fruits in the treatment of diseases of the respiratory system. He referred to raspberry wine as a "great cordial" capable of cleansing the blood, comforting the heart, easing pains in the stomach, dispelling vapors from the brain, causing free breathing, preventing pestilential air and removing obstructions from the lungs. The wine of blackberries is particularly helpful in the prevention of infection from "pestilential airs"; and the wine of English figs, particularly appropriate to defects of the lungs and in the treatment of dyspepsia and inflammations. In recent times Martinet[14] prescribes various wines and cognac for the treatment of many pulmonary ailments including bronchitis, bronchopneumonia, asthma and pulmonary congestion. Spilsbury[15] reports, "I have for several years watched the beneficial use of wine in acute bronchitis and from extensive experience and observation, am warranted in giving corroborative testimony relative to the use of wine and brandy administered in small doses." Cruchet[16] goes even further to state, "One knows that in our day the mortality from grippe is infinitely less among wine drinkers." Jager[17] prescribes warm, sweet wine as a preventive and abortive in acute respiratory infections and influenza, especially during the chill. When cardiac embarrassment and failure are present in lobar pneumonia, Young and Beaumont[18] advise that small doses of tincture of digitalis may be given with potassium iodide or brandy.

At the beginning of the 20th century, it was customary to use alcoholic beverages in the treatment of any respiratory disease. At present alcoholic beverages are, in general, contraindicated in the acute phases of respiratory diseases unless there is some especial indication for their administration. However, in convalescence from pneumonia as well as from any other severe and debilitating disease the use of wine is highly recommended.[19] Judiciously administered, it improves the appetite and promotes a feeling of general well-being.

Summarizing, we may conclude that alcohol in moderation exerts a minor but appreciable stimulatory effect on pulmonary ventilation. It produces a slight increase in the total volume of air passing through the lungs and in the amount of oxygen absorbed from the alveolar epithelium. Wines and brandies—which contain large amounts of esters—exert a more pronounced effect upon the respiratory mechanism than ethyl alcohol or simple wines.

Two generalizations may be drawn from the accumulated experimental data on the effects of alcohol on the respiratory system: (*1*) that the alcohol level of blood in the alveolar capillaries is rapidly equilibrated with that of the systemic circulation during forced ventilation; and (*2*) that although the rate of excretion of alcohol appears to be increased during the inhalation of oxygen and carbon dioxide mixtures, it rapidly returns to its former level following the period of increased ventilation.

The apparent decrease in the concentration of alcohol in the blood during forced ventilation induced by mixtures of carbon dioxide-oxygen returns to its former level following cessation of hyperventilation. It is assumed that this phenomenon is subject to and dominated by the concentration of alcohol in the tissues. Furthermore, the experimental studies indicate that the ingestion of alcohol fails to effect any specific dynamic changes in the basal metabolic rate.

The therapeutic use of wine in acute respiratory infections dates back to the ancients. In modern times it has proven effective in the treatment of bronchitis, bronchopneumonia, asthma and other allied affections of the lungs. Warm wine is prescribed during the period of chilling in influenza and in other respiratory infections. A glass of wine taken at bedtime will often forestall a cold by acting as a sudorific. Alcoholic beverages must be used judiciously during the acute phase of the pneumonias. However, as in any other debilitating disease, they are highly recommended during the period of convalescence.

VI. *The Action of Wine upon the Cardiovascular System*

‖‖‖

"Wine," wrote the 13th-century physician, Arnald of Villanova, "strengthens by its own virtue the substance of the heart."[1] In the intervening centuries, alcohol has won recognition as a powerful stimulant in the treatment of diseases of the cardiovascular system. According to Moerchen,[2] the stimulating effect of wine has been proven scientifically, and a specific cardiovascular therapeutic element has been recovered from cognac.

Pardee[3] warns that there is danger "of giving too little and failing to get stimulation of the heart or of giving too much and causing depression." However, "alcohol is an excellent analgesic, relieving pain or discomfort or the sense of shortness of breath, making the patient feel better and more comfortable, and often promoting a much-needed sleep. It may be used in this way in the acute infections or in chronic illnesses and competes with chloral hydrate, the bromides, luminal and similar drugs. Sometimes one, sometimes another will act best."

Pons and Broeckaert[4] state that the alcohol in wine can render incontestable service as a heart stimulant. Charcot, Llagnet, and Guillermin[5] agree that "generous wines" in fractionated doses act as stimulants in serious diseases of the heart. In those whose hearts are weak and in whom the pulse is feeble, Dontas[6] notes, good wine has an immediate

tonic action on the pulse and the coronary circulation.
In the treatment of endocarditis, Dieulafoy[7] recommends
Trousseau's wine: 1 tablespoon daily for 5 or 6 days:

White wine	7 pints
Alcohol (90 per cent)	17 ounces
Juniper berries	12 ounces
Acetate of potash	7 ounces
Digitalis leaves	2 ounces
Squill	1 ounce

This he describes as "a diuretic which does not exhaust the
kidney and a cardiac tonic which does not exhaust the
heart." Fitch[8] agrees with Sir Clifford Allbutt that in chronic
diseases of the heart a moderate glass of good claret, hock
or light sherry taken with the meal should serve as an
effective medicine and "suffice for cheerfulness" and that the
use of brandy in the cardiac failure which accompanies acute
disease is indicated.

The eminent 18th-century English physician, William
Heberden,[9] was the first to recognize and advocate the
beneficial effects of wine, cordials and cognac for the relief
of the pain of angina pectoris. The rapidity and effectiveness
with which alcohol relieves cardiac pain accounts for its widespread use in the treatment of this disease. Brooks[10] observed that in the treatment of angina pectoris the most
satisfactory results follow the regular administration of
wine with meals and at bedtime. Besides the purely chemical
effects of wine, it is in addition beneficial because of its unquestionable euphoric effects. This action is greatly to be
desired in angina pectoris because there is "no other condition in which depression, apprehension and anxiety of the
quiet periods almost equal the acute agony of the actual
paroxysms." Brooks also prescribes wine for the purpose
of mitigating, interrupting or aborting paroxysms of coronary artery spasm. He comments on the advisability of using
brandy and wines in heart disease in preference to other

forms of alcohol, and states that any alcoholic beverage is contraindicated when the primary cause of the heart ailment is gout. The beneficial action of wines, Clark[11] points out, is much greater than that of alcohol alone . . . It is possible that these drinks contain substances other than alcohol which act as cardiac tonics. Both Stockton[12] and Bishop[13] attribute the relief of the pain of angina pectoris to vasodilatation of the coronary arteries. The same dilatation of the peripheral blood vessels is responsible for the sensation of warmth one feels following the ingestion of a pleasant alcoholic beverage.[14] Alcohol has been found to be efficacious in relieving the pain of severe forms of obliterative vascular disease. Cook and Brown[15] administered 0.5 cubic centimeters of alcohol per kilogram of body weight to a large group of patients afflicted with thromboangiitis obliterans, Raynaud's disease and arteriosclerosis with thrombosis. A study of the skin temperatures of their subjects indicated that in addition to its properties as a pain-relieving agent, alcohol is a more effective vascular dilator than acetyl choline.

As far back as 1870, Parkes and Wollowicz[16] studied the action of red Bordeaux wine on the human body. They found that when it was taken with dinner it substantially accelerated the frequency of the pulse and increased the work load of the heart. Later, Loeb[17] determined that minor concentrations of alcohol (0.13 to 0.3 per cent) added to the perfusate produced a noticeable stimulatory effect on the isolated mammalian heart. These observations were confirmed by Bachem[18] and ultimately by Dixon[19] who, using an elaborate heart-lung preparation, found that alcohol added to the perfusing solution resulted in a marked improvement in the stroke output. Continuing along the same lines, Sulzer and Cannan[20] noted that concentrations of 0.1 to 0.2 per cent alcohol in the perfusing fluid were also successful in increasing the coronary output. However, at a concentration of 1.0 per cent—an amount well beyond physiologic limits—the action of the heart was found to be decidedly impaired.

The Russian physician, Kootataladse,[21] isolated an amine from wine which exerts an effect upon the coronary circulation of the heart independent of the effect of alcohol. This substance, which is soluble in both alcohol and water, is not found in fresh grape juice. It apparently is a by-product of fermentation or vinification. When used in dilutions of 1:500,000, it increased the coronary flow and doubled the output of the isolated mammalian heart.

In the treatment of hypertension, alcohol often serves to alleviate the apprehension and general discomfort associated with this disease. Here again Brooks[10] advocates the use of wines in preference to the more concentrated types of alcoholic medicinal agents. Beverage alcohol should not be prescribed in cases of hypertension when etiologically a renal lesion is suspected and red blood cells appear in the urine. As far as can be ascertained, moderate amounts of alcohol have no effect on blood pressure. Cabot[22] and Lieb[23] administered alcohol to a group of hospitalized patients and noted no change whatsoever in the blood pressure readings. However, when changes do occur, they are always in the direction of a fall, not a rise.[24] McDowell[25] states that alcohol in therapeutic amounts reduces the venous pressure in man, an effect predictable from the general physiologic properties of this substance.

Clinically, the incidence of coronary thrombosis seems not to be increased by the intake of beverage alcohol. In fact, the incidence of the disease seems to be less among regular consumers of beverage alcohol than among nonusers. This clinical impression has been significantly stated and repeatedly confirmed.[22, 26]

It is alleged that the incidence of arteriosclerosis among those who consume alcohol is one-half that of a normal random population and only one-sixth that of a diabetic population. This phenomenon is attributed to the increased solubility of cholesterol in dilute solutions of alcohol. Eberhard[27] has demonstrated experimentally in rabbits that a diet high in cholesterol to which alcohol is added results in a higher blood cholesterol content than when the same diet is administered without alcohol. However, the cholesterol deposition in the liver and aorta is definitely lower in the group fed alcohol. Wilder[28] states that "it has never been proved that alcohol provokes arteriosclerosis, and because of its vasodilating action it may even be useful in cases of diabetic arteriosclerosis and diminished peripheral circulation."

In short, alcohol is accepted as an "effective stimulant" in the treatment of cardiovascular disease; and the beneficial action of wines appears to be greater than that of the more concentrated forms of alcoholic beverages. Both brandy and wines have proven to be of therapeutic value in:

(*1*) stimulating the coronary circulation in conditions characterized by depressed physiologic activity and in diseases of the heart which require immediate action;

(*2*) relieving the pain of angina pectoris and obliterative vascular diseases;

(*3*) increasing the stroke volume output of the heart: and

(*4*) alleviating the discomfort associated with hypertension and allied conditions in general.

Used in moderation, alcohol seems to have no effect upon the blood pressure. However, there are two circumstances under which its use is contraindicated: (*a*) when the heart condition is caused by gout, and (*b*) when hypertension acompanies active nephritis or its etiology presupposes a renal lesion. Finally, alcohol appears not to be a contributory factor in either coronary thrombosis or arteriosclerosis.

VII. The Action of Wine upon the Kidneys, and Its Use in Renal Disease

||||||||||||||||||||||||||||||||||||||||||||||||||||||||||||||||||||||||||||||||||||||||||||||||||||||||||||||||||||||||||||||||||||||||||||||||||||||||||||||||||||||||||||

The effect of alcohol on the kidneys and urinary tract has been under discussion for many years, particularly because Richard Bright[1] included over-indulgence in alcohol as an etiologic factor in nephritis. The impression, however, has not been confirmed either experimentally or clinically. Dickinson[2] was "very skeptical of the role of alcohol in the production of renal disease; he found that the incidence of diseased kidneys was no greater in those who died of delirium tremens than in those who died of accident, nor was it higher in those engaged in the liquor traffic than in persons with occupations less predisposing to intemperance." Both Fahr[3] and Fishberg[4] have amassed experimental and clinical data to illustrate that alcohol has no deleterious effect on the kidneys. After repeated administrations of alcohol to rabbits, Friedenwald[5] found no evidence that the pathologic changes of chronic Bright's disease had been satisfactorily attained. Similarly, MacNider[6] concluded that in normal dogs an inebriating amount of ethyl alcohol "is but slightly nephrotoxic" as measured by tests of renal function and routine urinalyses. In these experiments the kidneys appeared normal histologically. Bruger, Localio and Guthrie[7] studied the effect of alcohol and whisky in moderate doses on human subjects suffering from various forms of renal disease. They concluded that "alcohol or whisky has no deleterious effect on the kidneys of normal subjects nor does it aggravate the renal lesion in patients with acute or chronic glomerular nephritis." However, in patients with arteriosclerotic nephritis, transient hematuria and temporary diminution of renal function were observed.

Many contemporary authors, Wegelin,[8] Cohnheim and Marchand,[9] Ziegler and Horner[10] offer evidence that the regular consumption of alcohol does not impair the kidneys, and, furthermore, that the vascular bed of the kidneys under the influence of alcohol appears to be patulous. It would be in order to infer that insofar as the kidneys are concerned alcoholic beverages are diuretic. Widmark[11] observed that the concentration of alcohol in the urine is strikingly similar to that in the blood. Miles,[12] in observing the rate and rapidity of absorption and excretion of alcohol, concluded that "the percent of alcohol eliminated in the urine within two hours after ingestion is 1.2 to 1.6 of that ingested. The major part of the elimination occurs in this period provided the bladder is emptied two or three times." On the other hand, Haggard and Greenberg[13] found that "the concentration of alcohol in the urine bears no relation to the volume of urine secreted; the amount of alcohol eliminated through the kidneys, however, varies directly with the volume secreted. The percentage of the total amount of alcohol ingested that is lost through the kidneys depends, therefore, upon the amount of urine passed." On the basis of these findings they concluded that during a period of "sixteen hours following ingestion of alcohol from 2.1 to 4.3 per cent of the total amount is eliminated through the kidneys, the variation depending upon the rate of secretion of urine."

The essence of recent research on the diuretic effect of wine indicates that the diuretic action of white wine is greater than that of red wine;[14] that the diuretic response is greater in patients afflicted with acute and chronic diffuse glomerular nephritis than in persons with other renal diseases;[15] and that patients with renal insufficiency due to hypertension appear to be more sensitive to the diuretic action of wine than normal subjects.[16] Bastedo[17] ascribes the heightened diuretic effect to a secondary dilatation of the renal arterioles. This permits a greater flow of blood to the glomeruli and the resulting increase in urinary output is due to an increase of oxygen available to the glomeruli. In Bastedo's opinion, the increased intake of fluids is also an important factor. Carles[18] studied the diuretic effects of white wines and red wines with especial reference to the content of organic acids and their potassium salts. Although he admits that white wines are more diuretic than red wines, their differences cannot be attributed to their salt contents. Similar distinctions are also mentioned by Vincent,[19] Dougnac,[20] and Weissenbach.[21] According to Vincent, sweet wine owes its rapid diuretic effects to organic salts of potassium, particularly to the bitartrate which, in the course of its metabolism, is reduced to potassium carbonate, an effective diuretic.

In contrast, the effectiveness of red wine on renal excretion is attributed to tannin and its combination with other substances which enhance it as an astringent. These substances perhaps are responsible for the characteristic reactions of red wine. Mrak and Fessler[22] have shown that the presence of buffers in wine prevents the acidosis which ordinarily follows the ingestion of alcohol. They attribute this effect to the natural tartrates and phosphates contained in the grape which constitute a source of reserve alkali. Saywell,[23] in studying urinary acidity, found that the ingestion of grapes and their products decreased the excretion of ammonia and increased the urinary pH, the excretion of organic acids and alkaline reserve. Clouse,[24] in confirming these data, noted an increased output of organic acid (primarily uric and citric) and a greater total alkaline residue.

Oenotherapy is not always prescribed in kidney ailments

despite the fact that it is indicated more often than many
clinicians realize. Labbe[25] prescribed wine in the treatment
of nephritis and Manquat[26] stated that "if milk is not
tolerated in kidney disease, take a little light white wine."
Moderate amounts of wine are favored by Mosenthal,[27]
Van Noorden,[28] and Fishberg,[29] who agree that it enhances
the appetite and increases the receptiveness of the patient
to the prescribed diet which is often monotonous. During
the period of quiescence in Bright's disease, Dougnac[30]
recommends a small amount of wine diluted with alkaline
water. He also prescribes in renal lithiasis a wine of low
alcoholic content diluted with water.

The consensus, then, seems to be that alcohol in dilute
concentration does not have the injurious effect upon the
kidneys it was once thought to have. In addition, it has been
demonstrated that alcohol does not irritate the ureters or
bladder. White wine, which has a more pronounced diuretic
action, is of greater therapeutic value than red wine in this
particular field of medicine. It may be prescribed with
benefit in all types of nephritis excepting in renal insufficiency, especially that due to hypertension and in arteriosclerotic nephritis.[31] Lastly, wine may be used effectively
in renal disease as a preventive of acidosis and as an adjuvant to the alkaline reserve.

VIII. *The Action of Wine upon the Neuromuscular System*

‖‖

The literature of the world from Biblical times to the present day attests to the fact that mankind values wine for its influence upon both the mind and the physique. Of all the organs of the body, the one which apparently responds most sensitively to wine is the human brain.

In Billings' symposium,[1] the following statement occurs: "One need not be skilled in psychology to note the effects of moderate quantities of wine at social gatherings. The speech and bearing of men, the play of features, all bear witness to its power. Restraints are removed, too acute sensibilities are blunted, little acerbities are smoothed down, ideas and mental images follow each other with greater rapidity, a 'cerebral sense of richness,' and lastly a condition of euphoria, a more serene state of consciousness, ensues."

Granted that alcohol in the form of wine effects psychologic changes, the question is whether it acts as a stimulant or a sedative. Certainly a superficial observation would lead one to infer that alcohol is a cerebral stimulant. However, the preponderance of opinion does not bear out this conclusion. Kraepelin[2] is one of the few exceptions. On the basis of numerous psychologic experiments, he concludes that "in the early stages of its action alcohol truly stimulates the motor functions of the brain; that a state of mental exhilaration, of 'motor excitability,' may coexist with undiminished power of perception and judgment."

On the other hand, pharmacologists of high repute, notably Mitscherlich and Schmiedeberg,[3] emphatically hold that even in moderation alcohol is not a cerebral stimulant. Some functions of the brain, Schmiedeberg declares, are weakened or immobilized before others, and one of the first effects is loss of restraint. The apparent "excitement" following the consumption of alcohol is, in reality, the after-effect of a release of the inhibitory control or a lack of psychic coordination. The proponents of this hypothesis look upon alcohol as a sedative or narcotic. They claim that its stimulating effect is deceptive and that even the early phenomena mentioned by Kraepelin are due to depression of cerebral function.

Moerchen[4] believed that wine, because of its slightly narcotizing effect and the influence it exerts on the regulatory mechanism of the circulation, "has greater value as a means of moral and nervous relaxation than any other alcoholic drink." In a study of the sedative action of alcohol, Mullin, Kleitman and Cooperman[5] recorded the movements of sleepers who earlier had taken an amount of alcohol equivalent in concentration to a glass of port. They found that the tossing movements of light sleepers definitely decreased during the first half of the night. In another study[6] of the sedative action of alcohol on the central nervous system, it was observed that dilute concentrations slightly increased the electrical excitability of the hypothalamus with resultant stimulation whereas larger doses caused depression. On one point there is no doubt; at least one-third ounce of alcohol must be taken before the trained observer can detect "even the most insignificant departure from the normal course of brain and nerve processes."[7] Larger amounts are necessary before alcohol brings a flush to the skin and accelerates the rate of the pulse and respiration. In order to produce even a slight increase in oxygen intake, 20 to 30 cubic centimeters of alcohol are required—an equivalent, in terms of table wine, of approximately seven to ten ounces.

Alcohol in the form of wine is particularly recommended for certain types, such as nervous persons past middle age for whom it "may be absolutely beneficial."[8] On the battlefield where the French consider it "the soul of the soldier," wine "activates circulation, increases muscular energy and resists fatigue."[9] (Eylaud and Macard[10] suggest that the soldier's weight and load determine the amount of wine to be included in his alimentary ration.) In short, Bonguiod[11] states, the use of wine "should coincide with an active life." For the laborer who uses his muscles, it even may be a physiologic necessity![12]

Vernon[13] and his associates have provided extensive experimental evidence concerning the action of alcohol on neuromuscular coordination in typing, working an adding machine and in pricking a target. A summary of the effects of alcohol on the accuracy and speed of these operations includes the following points:

(1) For typists and adding machine operators: alcohol produced the same effect on both kinds of workers. In some subjects, moderate amounts of alcoholic beverages taken with food produced no measurable reaction. However, alcohol taken on an empty stomach was found to be twice as active as when imbibed with food. In the foodless experiments, one subject made 88 per cent more typing mistakes after 11.2 cubic centimeters of alcohol; another made 156 per cent more after 22 cubic centimeters of alcohol; a third increased his adding machine errors 74 per cent after 19.4 cubic centimeters of alcohol.

(2) For target practice: rows of dots on squared paper, fixed vertically at arm's length, were pricked at three-minute intervals before and after the consumption of alcohol. Before taking alcohol, the average distance between the prick and the center of the target was 1.8 millimeters; after taking

30 cubic centimeters of alcohol, the target-pricking errors increased 12 per cent; and after 37.5 cubic centimeters, 43 per cent. They continued to increase in arithmetical progression with augmented doses of alcohol until with 66 cubic centimeters the errors were increased to 132 per cent above normal. The influence of alcohol on the production of errors was directly proportional to the quantity ingested and to the complexity of the manipulative procedures involved.

As in any other chemical compound representing a combination of carbon, hydrogen and oxygen, and classified as carbohydrate, alcohol is oxidized in the body to yield energy. Although little is known about the effects of small amounts of alcohol on the muscles (considered apart from the nervous system), this substance has not been found to be as "practicable a source of energy for prolonged physical labor as equivalent amounts of food proper."[14] Furthermore, it also has been fairly well established that increased muscular exertion does not increase the rate of combustion of ingested alcohol.[15]

Considerable research has been done on the influence of alcohol on voluntary muscular effort, most of it on the employment of certain groups of muscles rather than on the reaction of all the muscles (such as would be involved in manual labor). The consensus is that "small quantities of alcohol have but a slight and temporary stimulating action on voluntary work; and all are agreed that any considerable quantity, say two ounces of absolute alcohol (the amount assumed to be oxidized in 24 hours, with only the usual physiological loss by escape through the excretory channels), lowers the ability to do muscular work."[16] Lombard[17] found that in human subjects, small quantities of claret increased the amount of muscular work for a period of only one hour after its ingestion.

Destree's[18] researches took into account the element of muscular fatigue after the ingestion of alcohol, and led him to the following conclusions:

(*a*) that the same stimulating effect is obtained when muscles are vigorous as when they are exhausted;

(*b*) that the stimulating effect is noticeable immediately after the administration of alcohol, but lasts only briefly;

(*c*) that this temporary stimulation is always followed by depression. "In about half an hour after the administration of the alcohol the work done reaches a minimum." Additional amounts exert only a slight stimulating action; and

(*d*) that the subsequent depression overbalances the original stimulation to the point that the total amount of work accomplished with alcohol is less than that done without it.

Schumberg[19] found alcohol to be "devoid of a direct dynamogenic power for muscular tissue." His conclusions were of significance because they were based upon results of reactions of the entire body engaged in hard labor rather than on any restricted group of muscles. Scheffer[20] carried on an even more extensive series of experiments which illustrated the increase in voluntary work following the ingestion of alcohol and the subsequent decrease, to a point below normal, as soon as the stimulatory effects were worn off. His results were obtained from "three series of experiments, in the first of which the tests were begun immediately after taking the alcohol; in the second fifteen minutes after the alcohol was taken. In the third series of tests the alcohol was taken thirty minutes before the experiments were begun, and in this series the mechanical labor performed was 5.61 per cent. less in amount than the experiments without alcohol. In the first series there was a gain of 5.81 per cent. in the work done as estimated in kilogrammetres, in the second series the gain amounted to 8.7 per cent. The results of the third series show very clearly how rapidly the fatiguing effects of alcohol come on, and how much they tend to repress the output of energy by the muscle substance." Although admitting that "alcohol undoubtedly enables men to push themselves for a short time beyond the limit which nature otherwise would have imposed on them," Cabot,[21] in confirming Scheffer's findings, reports that in his experiments the power of voluntary muscular movement increased about 7 per cent for the first half hour after taking alcohol and was followed by a decrease to about 5 per cent below normal. Auguet[22] encourages the discreet consumption of wine to increase the output of the human machine even though its effects are temporary. In his opinion, good wine (preferably red wine) complements the basic ration of energy food. "It gives to the worker or athlete, the factor of stimulation necessary for his neuromuscular tone. Better than sugar—and less waste to the organism—it permits the prolongation of effort, and increases the output from 15 per cent to 20 per cent."

Whatever its effect on muscular power, there is no question that the general weariness experienced by the average person at the end of the day diminishes after a glass of wholesome wine. Jaillet[23] advised the moderate use of alcohol for just this purpose, adding that it should be "in the form of wine and taken with the meal." Mauriac,[24] Fitch,[25] Loeper and Alquier,[26] and Cuvier[27] are among the later authorities who agree that in general wine exerts a restorative action on those exhausted by fatigue. Cazalis,[28] our contemporary, says "for patients over-worked, fatigued, neurasthenic, a little wine with meals favorably influences the nervous system." However, none of the moderns is as ingenious as a 19th-century practitioner, Kitchiner, who advised that "feeble persons, subject to such sudden attacks (exhaustion) should always travel armed with a pocket pistol charged with a couple of glasses of white wine."[29]

In consideration of the use of wine in "nervous shock-collapse," Anstie[30] distinguishes between two types of collapse. In his opinion, stimulants of any kind are contraindicated in the state of "shock depression" that begins with a sudden rigor, followed by mild hysteria. The use of wine or brandy is therapeutically sound, he states, only in cases of "true shock-collapse" where the object is to "rouse the attention of the brain." For this purpose, he considers the strongest stimulants in concentrated form the best: one ounce of half-and-half brandy and water every fifteen minutes. "A very few doses," he adds, "are all that are useful; the rest of the work must be done by such stimulations as surface-heat, friction &c., and advantage must be taken of the earliest opportunity to administer food, if the patient be in a state of fast."

In the past, alcohol was considered to be the causative factor of peripheral neuritis, pellagra, certain encephalopathies, and Wernicke's disease. The modern clinicians[31] agree with Minot, Strauss and Cobb[32] that these ailments stem from vitamin deficiencies and bear only an oblique relation to alcohol. It is now held that an exclusive diet of alcoholic beverages will cause deficiency disease in much the same way as a diet composed entirely of any other single item.[33] Campbell and Biggart[34] point out that this mechanism of dietary deficiency is undoubtedly responsible for many of the so-called alcoholic psychoses. Experiments have been performed to determine the effect of alcohol in polyneuropathy. Using thiamine-deficient rats, Lowry and his co-workers[35] noted that their data did not support the assumption that the ingestion of alcohol increases the thiamine requirement. Furthermore, they proved that the neurologic manifestations of thiamine deficiency could be prevented or alleviated by the administration of thiamine regardless of the presence or absence of alcohol.

In many diseases of the neuromuscular system, the use of alcohol is generally inadvisable. There are, however, notable exceptions. Among these are certain chronic neuroses and neuralgias relatively common in the later decades of life. Anstie[36] states that "the misery which these neuralgias inflict, and the extent to which they shatter the system, is deplorable under the best of circumstances; and we need every helpful adjunct we can get. The reflex irritation which the disease sets up is often fatal at once to appetite and to sleep; and wine is the true remedy for this part of the mischief." In conclusion, he adds that "the older the wine, the more endowed with ethereal ingredients, the more effective it is for this purpose." Another exception, according to Anstie, is the type of chorea which occurs in "naturally feeble and anaemic patients, especially when the attack has been precipitated by severe emotional shock." An instance where "the value of the potent and also highly etherised wines can hardly be over-rated, is the acute form of chorea which threatens life, and which in so many instances does prove fatal. Here there is very often a tolerance for large doses which is extraordinary, and so long as we keep below the line of narcotism and administer the stimulant with regularity and watchfulness, there is no need for timidity as to quantity; the danger is pressing, and a very large total daily allowance may be absolutely necessary." In prescribing white wines for the asthenic and melancholic, Eylaud[37] observes that the ethers in wine play an important role "from the point of view of their effect on the nerve centers."

Trapp and Schube[38] used alcohol as a diagnostic agent in order to study the intellectual and emotional responses in mental illness. A 40 per cent solution of ethyl alcohol was administered by stomach tube in fractional doses. An initial dose of 30 cubic centimeters was given, followed by a small quantity of water as a flushing agent. At four-minute intervals extra doses of 15 cubic centimeters were administered in a similar manner until a maximum of 120 cubic centimeters was given. The last four doses were administered at ten-minute intervals for a final total dose of 180 cubic centimeters. The patients were observed and questioned before, during and after the procedure. Alcohol was found to be of value in the diagnosis of psychoses in which mutism conceals the true nature of the emotional content; in differentiating the varieties of stupor; and in probing the intellectual level underlying certain depressive states. Trapp and Schube concluded, however, that alcohol is of no permanent therapeutic value in the treatment of mental illness.

Alexandre and Aparici[39] found wine to be a tonic of immediate effect in neurasthenia, "stimulating the nervous system and favoring oxidation." Weissenbach[40] also speaks of the tonic action of wine on the neuromuscular system. One of the illnesses in which it has proven most effective is severe Parkinsonism. Fabing and Zeligs[41] have achieved eminently satisfactory results from the use of an extract of Bulgarian belladonna root suspended in white table wine.

It is apparent from the preceding discussion that because of the sedative effect wine exerts on the cerebral processes, it is probably of greater value as a means of relaxation than any other alcoholic beverage. It may be concluded that moderate amounts of alcohol are without appreciable effect on manual labor requiring skill and delicacy of muscular control, but that above a certain limit the increasing lack of neuromuscular coordination varies directly with the amount of alcohol consumed and indirectly with the tolerance of the individual. Furthermore, it may be stated that food delays the absorption of alcohol. As for muscular exertion, alcohol acts as a brief but temporary stimulant. The consensus is that fatigue is not a factor, nor does the increased exertion affect the rate of combustion of the ingested alcohol. However, the fatigue experienced by the average person at the end of an arduous day is pleasantly relieved by a glass of wine taken with the evening meal.

The role of alcohol in the treatment of diseases of the neuromuscular system is conditioned by opinion. In nervous shock, wine and brandy may be beneficial in the treatment of the collapse but not the depression. They have proven to be of genuine therapeutic value in the treatment of the chronic neuroses common to later life. In general, it may be said that alcohol is a "revivifying remedy," one that "rejoices the heart of man, and revives the nervous system when it is exhausted."[42]

IX. *The Use of Wine in Acute Infectious Diseases*

||||||||||||||||||||||||||||||||||||||||||||||||||||||||||||||||||||||||||||||||||||||||||||||||||||||||||||||||||||||||||||||||||||||||||||||||||||||||||||||||||||||||||||||

Wine, as an antiseptic, is older than Hippocratic medicine, whereas its use to combat infectious diseases dates from a later generation. In French literature, great importance has been attributed to the apparent bacteriostatic action of wine on the disease-producting bacteria which attack the bowel, particularly the typhoid-paratyphoid group. Hippocrates prescribed wine in the treatment of wounds, and St. Luke echoed this advice. Dougnac[1] mentions the application of aromatic wine to heal external ulcers and recommends its use in gargles and strong douches.

Anstie,[2] 19th-century physician and author of a delightful, informative monograph on oenotherapy, advocates moderate quantities of wine in both febrile and nonfebrile diseases. In fevers it is his opinion that the use of alcohol is indicated by the following combination of factors: (*a*) a high temperature; (*b*) delirium or any other evidence of nervous prostration; (*c*) tachycardias, especially those which are dichrotic, and irregularities in which the unrhythmic beat reflects rapid and irregular changes in the force and action of the heart. In such cases, the pharmacologic value of wine is due largely to its ethereal constituents and its low alcoholic content. In regard to these components of wine, Anstie remarks "the ethereal constituents of wine have a special value in the later stages of severe febrile disease with great exhaustion of the heart, especially when combined with sleeplessness. On the other hand, a low alcoholic strength of wine, together with the presence of carbonic acid, as in finer effervescing wines, is particularly useful in cases where the violence of the fever, the nervous prostration, and the derangement of digestion are out of proportion to the gravity of the case as regards danger to life and continuous destruction of tissue."[3] Anstie further recommends highly etherized wines for acute delirium. "Sometimes a very few glasses," he observes, "will suffice to restore the patient to a condition in which he becomes willing to take those supplies of food"[4] needed for his safety.

Light, effervescent wines, as opposed to the strongly alcoholized varieties, are recommended in the treatment of the inflammatory phases of most contagious diseases. In the treatment of catarrhal fevers and inflammations, one is admonished to choose wines with great care; they should not contain more than 6 or 7 per cent absolute alcohol and should be very dry.[5] Shaw[6] interjects a precautionary note. "I do not say that this excellent liquor should be indiscriminately given in all kinds of fevers, and particularly in such as are inflammatory—but in the worst kind of fevers attended with a slow pulse, great heaviness, stupor, retching, deliria, etc., 'tis the most sovereign remedy hitherto made use of."

In the class of inflammatory infections chiefly represented by pneumonia and bronchitis of the aged, and especially if unaccompanied by fever, the victims likewise benefit from the therapeutic action of wine. Anstie also was impressed by the effect of wines on intestinal ailments, particularly the obstinate catarrhal diarrheas so common in the England of his time. Sir William Osler[7] shared Anstie's respect for the beneficial effect of wine when he stated, "I should be sorry to give up its use in the severe form of enteric and pneumonic fevers." In substantiation of these statements, Himwich[8] has demonstrated that with the administration of alcohol in moderate concentrations, it is not unlikely that the tissues remove less dextrose from the blood, indicating that alcohol, a food substitute, by supplying energy to the body has spared its carbohydrate stores. Fantus[9] has amplified this observation. Alcohol, he notes, is oxidized more rapidly and more completely by a febrile person than by that same person under conditions of normal body temperature. Its food value, he concludes, might be of consideration, particularly in cases where digestion is impaired. The glycogen-sparing effect of discriminate amounts of alcohol might be of substantial aid to the over-burdened liver of the debilitated febrile patient.

Experimentally, Soresi[10] administered wine by proctoclysis to a group of hospitalized pneumonia patients, all of whom responded well to this adjunctive form of treatment. He reported that their recovery was speedier and easier than that of patients who had not received wine by this novel means.

As long ago as 1838, Royer-Collard[11] prescribed wine in certain forms of typhus which he characterized as presenting pronounced adynamic symptoms with or without nervous exhaustion and/or a fever which was "far from being the expression of a true state of reaction."

Brichteteau[12] reported that wine is always well-tolerated by the subject of typhoid fever—the abdominal symptoms are modified; diarrhea, gurgling and meteorism diminish; the humidity of the tongue is restored; thirst is appeased; the skin reacquires its normal moisture; sleep becomes both peaceful and refreshing; and the alvine functions become regular. Therefore, "one cannot recommend the use of wine too highly in typhoid fever." Anstie[13] also acknowledges the salutary effect of wine on the victims of typhoid. Wetmore[14] records that "claret, mixed with the juice of lemon or limes is useful in preventing the evil effects of typhoid infection."

Wine as a therapeutic aid in epidemics is mentioned by Mauriac,[15] who advises that in times of cholera or typhoid it is wise to drink only pure wine or wine diluted with boiled water, and to abstain completely from other forms of alcohol. Dougnac[16] makes the point that the incidence of typhoid in the wine-drinking regions of France is lower generally than in those parts of the country where the beverage is less easily available. In view of the low reputation French drinking water enjoys, perhaps the natives have taken to wine consumption in intestinal self-defense.

In our own time, Violle and Rosé[17] studied the incidence of typhoid in Marseille and learned that many of the inhabitants found the taste of chlorine so obnoxious that they preferred to risk illness rather than take a mixture of the germicidal Javel solution with their drinking water. They suggested a different solution, namely: 50 cubic centimeters of red wine per liter of chlorinated water. This proved to be a satisfactory substitute. It removed the excess chlorine, and was palatable. Above all, it acted "as a mild disinfectant." Certainly there is no doubt that wine exerts a "remarkable effect" even on contaminated water. "Pure, it does not spare bacilli." Diluted with greatly polluted water (20,000 *E. coli* per liter) "it still controls victoriously."[18] In a careful series of laboratory researches on the bactericidal power of wine on bacilli of the dysentery group, Remlinger and Bailly[19] concluded that ordinary wines exert a bactericidal effect on the bacilli of dysentery similar to that which they exert on typhoid bacilli. Remlinger and Bailly acknowledge the bactericidal role of tannins and ethers but are unable, because of lack of data, to assign the mechanism of action which each exerts. Dietze,[20] on the other hand, maintains that the organic acid of wine adds to the germicidal power of the alcohol. The distinct germicidal power exerted by wine of low alcoholic content is due, he contends, to the favorable cooperation of alcohol and acid.

There is yet another infectious disease which responds to alcohol in the form of wine. The effectiveness of the light acid wines in preventing malaria among the inhabitants of marshy and other fever-stricken districts has been recognized fully, especially in the lowlands of France about the mouth of the Rhone.[21] An American university professor, F. T. Bioletti[22] cites a personal experience in corroboration of the hypothesis that wines effectively ward off disease. He spent six months in a malaria-ridden district with three groups of laborers. One included Irishmen, Germans and Negroes; another, Chinese; and a third was made up entirely of Frenchmen. Those laborers in the first two groups, who drank beer and whisky, suffered severe, often fatal attacks of malaria. Among the sixty Frenchmen who drank wine (seldom, if ever, to excess) there was only one case of malaria during the entire season.

Observations of Beckers,[23] made on French soldiers during World War I, indicate that wine may be a factor in susceptibility to minor infections. In the divisions of the French army where the consumption of wine was unrestricted, he noted that infection from small cuts and abrasions was insignificant when compared with the incidence of infection in those divisions where the use of wine was definitely circumscribed.

The investigations of McNaught and Pierce[24] concerning the effect of alcohol in trichinosis are significant. *In vitro* studies and experimentation on rats led them to these conclusions: (*1*) although a concentration of 25 per cent ethyl alcohol has little direct action on free trichinella larvae, concentrations as low as 9 per cent interfere with the digestive liberation of encysted larvae; and (*2*) a single dose of alcohol given to rats simultaneously with trichinous meat reduces by 80 per cent the number of trichinella encysting in the muscles. (This is due to the digestive interference described above.) However, when taken in large quantities over a period of many weeks—and during maturation, larval bearing, migrating and encysting stages of the parasites—there is no protection.

Several conclusions may be drawn from the preceding discussion. It is to be noted, for instance, that the ethereal constituents of wine and its low alcoholic content make it particularly suitable for use in both febrile and nonfebrile infections. These include catarrhal fevers and inflammations, intestinal disorders, pneumonia and bronchitis of the aged, typhoid, malaria and dysentery.

Several studies indicate that white wine is more powerful than red wine in its bactericidal effect on typhoid and dysentery bacilli. The therapeutic role of tannins and ethers is yet to be evaluated experimentally; however, there is no doubt that the germicidal power of wine is due to the combination of alcohol and other organic substances. Finally, it has been demonstrated that concentrations of alcohol as low as 9 per cent interfere with the digestive liberation of encysted trichinella.

X. *The Use of Wine in Diabetes Mellitus*

||||||||||||||||||||||||||||||||||||||||||||||||||||||||||||||||||||||||||||||||||||||||||||||||||||||||||||||||||||||||||||||||||||||||||||||||||||||||||||

Wine occupies a valuable position in the diet of the diabetic both under the present-day and pre-insulin methods of treatment. Prior to the advent of insulin, energy foods that could be utilized without burdening the pancreas or exaggerating its deficiency were of tremendous importance. Wine was then, as it is now, preferred as a source of beverage alcohol because of its moderate concentration and because of the fact that drinkers of wine are temperate. When the diabetic takes wine regularly in prescribed quantities with his meals, it serves as an excellent and predictable source of extra calories and does not require insulin for its assimilation.

The pioneer researches of Zuntz and Magnus-Levy,[1] done in 1891, demonstrate that alcohol does not lessen the utilization of food by the body, an observation of paramount importance, especially in the dietotherapy of diabetes. Atwater and Benedict[2] demonstrated that the coefficient of availability of alcohol is 98 per cent; that the potential energy of alcohol is transformed completely into kinetic energy either in the form of heat or of muscular work; and that alcohol protects body fat and protein. Furthermore, they emphasized the point that the alimentary digestion of alcohol does not interfere with the absorption of other foods, but in certain cases increases the efficiency of the absorption.

Benedict and Török[3] and later Neubauer[4] showed that

wine facilitates the oxidative processes in diabetics and enables them to burn carbohydrates with a decrease in glycosuria and acetonuria. From the food standpoint, alcohol has the advantage that it is perhaps the most readily oxidizable food substance with the possible exception of sugar. It is not only an efficient producer of energy, a sparer of fats and proteins, but it may supply up to 30 or 40 per cent of the caloric requirement of the body. It is not convertible into glucose or fatty acids and is therefore neither ketogenic nor antiketogenic. In view of these facts and from the standpoint of food, it is a valuable adjunct in the dietotherapy of diabetes mellitus.

Diner,[5] Gavrila and Sparchez,[6] Kolta[7] and Soula and Baisset[8] found significant decreases in the blood sugar levels of diabetics after ingestion of small amounts of alcohol. Experimental proof of these observations is provided by Burge[9] who concluded that "the administration of alcohol to diabetics is helpful because it stimulates the liver to an increased output of catalase which is carried by the blood to the tissues where it facilitates the oxidative processes with resulting increased oxidation of sugar and decreased acidosis." In a recent study, Tennent[10] found the blood sugar level of the normal human being to be unaffected by ingestion of moderate amounts of alcohol. Wiley[11] points out that the caloric value of alcohol at seven calories per gram is midway between that of protein and fat, and Porter[12] shows that these calories are ready and completely available as food without the "expenditure of digestive energy." Southgate[13] notes, as have many others, that the peak blood alcohol level when alcohol is taken with the meals is lower than that when it is taken without food.

Weissenbach[14] and his associates consider the use of alcohol in the form of wine as most effective in the treatment of diabetes mellitus. For the diabetic, wine continues to fulfill a significant function by satisfying caloric needs without aggravating the metabolic disturbance which is the basis of the disease; by supplying a pleasant aliment, it makes the restrictions of a Spartan diet less objectionable. When insulin resistance is encountered, dry wine becomes an even more important adjunct to the diet since it is an element in maintaining the nutritive balance without the necessity of insulin, especially in patients who suffer from low carbohydrate tolerance.

The limitation of the diet of the diabetic imposes a severe psychologic restriction on the patient, but it also imposes a moral obligation on the physician. In regard to diet in general, Lord Horder[15] states that "not upon how meagre a diet a patient can live, but upon what sort of a diet he can live most efficiently, should be the physician's guiding principle in ordering a patient's regimen. Neglect of this rule sometimes leads to anomalies to which either patient or doctor may be blinded by sentiment." On the other hand, Joslin[16] states that in no disease would the use of alcohol appear to be more beneficial or more justifiable, yet he does not prescribe it for personal reasons. Mellanby[17] states that in severe cases where the diet is markedly restricted from the point of view of energy, alcohol can be utilized as a useful adjunct for supplying energy without influencing the blood sugar level or producing glycosuria. In prescribing alcoholic beverages for energy purposes in the diabetic diet, many authorities judge the quantity to be given on the basis of the individual caloric tolerance of the subject. Alcoholic beverages taken in amounts greater than the tolerance of the individual may precipitate a return of glycosuria and other symptoms of active diabetes. In other words, the caloric tolerance which is limited in diabetics should determine the total daily quantity of alcohol they may use with safety. On this point, Mellanby and co-workers determined "the amount of alcohol the diabetic patient could oxidize each hour, and then gave this quantity hourly throughout the day," the quantity varying with the body weight, bodily activity and the metabolic equivalent of the person. "The alcohol burnt

COMPOSITION AND ENERGY VALUE OF WINES FOR THE CALCULATED DIET

Type of Wine	Alcohol gms/100 cc.	Extract gms/100 cc.	Reducing Sugar gms/100 cc.	Calories (Cals/100 cc.)*
TABLE WINES				
Red (California)				
Barbera	12.5	2.9	0.17	99.1
Burgundy	12.3	2.9	0.20	97.7
Cabernet	12.8	2.9	0.16	101.2
Chianti	12.7	2.8	0.12	100.1
Claret	12.1	3.1	0.33	97.1
Zinfandel	12.7	2.8	0.18	100.1
Red (French)				
Burgundy	{11.4 {13.1	{2.1 {2.8	{0.18 {0.24	{88.2 {102.9
Bordeaux	10.2	2.4	0.23	81.0
White (California)				
Chablis	11.6	2.3	0.21	90.4
Riesling	11.8	2.3	0.13	91.8
Sauterne (dry)	11.8	2.3	0.17	91.8
Sauterne	12.0	2.6	0.5	94.4
Sauterne (sweet)	12.3	4.6	2.15	115.1

White (French)				
Chablis	11.4	2.2	0.24	88.6
Sauternes	{12.9, 14.0}	{5.1, 8.1}	{3.33, 5.23}	{124.0, 151.3}
White (German)				
Rhine	10.1	2.9	0.23	82.3
Moselle	9.2	2.3	0.20	73.6
SPARKLING WINES (DRY)				
Champagne (California)	13.4	4.9	0.09	113.4
Champagne (French)	13.6	11.1	0.94	139.4
Burgundy (California)	11.7	4.7	1.99	108.7
Pink (California)	11.6	4.1	1.52	103.7
MISCELLANEOUS WINES				
Dry Sherry (California)	19.8	4.7	2.46	167.2
Dry Sherry (Spanish)	17.4	5.1	2.9	153.8
Vermouth (French)	16.9	7.0	4.5	164.3
Vermouth (Italian)	15.9	17.4	15.4	242.5

*When the amount of reducing sugar was less than 0.5 gm/100 cc., the number of calories it supplied to the total caloric content was ignored.

up by the average diabetic is of the order of 7 to 10 ccm. an hour." The use of alcoholic beverages in this manner is most effective in the treatment of the severe diabetic because it does not produce toxic symptoms nor increase the level of sugar in the blood. Furthermore, it allows the diabetic to live a more active and hence more normal life. In regard to the therapeutic effect of alcohol and especially the prevention of arteriosclerosis in the diabetic, Leary[18] states that in older patients alcohol, used intelligently, can be expected perhaps to delay the onset of arteriosclerosis and provide energy for a more useful life.

In the consideration of wine as food in the dietary formula of the diabetic, it is important to note that the type prescribed determines the extent of its beneficial action. Williamson[19] states that although wines may be rich in alcohol, those "which contain a large quantity of sugar must be avoided, but if the percentage of sugar is very small they may be permitted. Many old wines contain only a trace of sugar, and, as a rule, the older the wine the more suitable it is for diabetic patients; new wines should generally be avoided."

In "Dietetics for the Clinician," Bridges[20] devotes considerable space to the composition and fuel values of wines, which in general gives the essence of the problem as he found it. Recent analyses demonstrate that the alcohol and extract contents of present day wines are greater and their carbohydrate contents less than the values given by Bridges. For practical purposes a list of wines (see pp. 98 and 99) and their composition is given as a dietetic guide for the diabetic regimen. In general the carbohydrate content of the dry table wines can be ignored; however, the caloric value of the wine should be taken into consideration in the final expression of the diabetic diet.

Although wine is useful in diabetes regardless of the character or gravity of the condition, it is particularly effective in the diabetic difficult to control because of ketosis or wasting. In the majority of such cases, Weissenbach and his associates[21] recommend the addition of 1 liter of wine to the regimen because it reduces the need for large doses of insulin, or it may make the use of "insulin therapy unnecessary." The observations of the older clinicians must not be discarded too hastily. In a symposium delivered at the Royal Society of Medicine before the discovery of insulin, one of the participants commented on the large number of diabetics in whom the maximum diet represented an allowance of but 20 calories per kilogram per day, an amount less than one-half that necessary for the maintenance of life and energy at normal levels. "It is to these," he concluded, "that in my opinion alcohol is essential."[22]

In view of this important problem, a summary of the particular advantages of using alcoholic beverages in the dietetic regimen of the diabetic might include the following points: first, the fact that although alcohol is considered a substitute for carbohydrate it does not become converted into sugar during its metabolism. On the contrary, it decreases the excretion of sugar. In addition, it spares the body protein and fat and depresses the blood sugar level. The vitamin B content present in wine acts as an adjunct to the "glycolytic enzymes," often deficient in diabetes mellitus.[23] As a stomachic, alcohol accelerates the rate of absorption of glucose, and by stimulating the flow of pancreatic juices, it facilitates the assimilation of fats. To quote Lepine,[24] "it assists digestion and does not increase glycosuria." Jager[25] observes that "in acidosis, wine improves the utilization of nitrogenous matter and perhaps it esterifies through its alcohol, a certain amount of acids." Lastly, "through its diuretic power . . . [it] favors the elimination of waste."

As far as can be determined, moderate amounts of alcoholic beverages, low in sugar content, especially if the sugar be levulose or D-fructose[26] as in wine, may be included in the alimentary regimen throughout the evolution of diabetes mellitus, from the most benign form to the final stages with or without acidosis. In conclusion, alcoholic beverages assist in maintaining and sustaining energy and augmenting the consciousness of well-being that plays such an important part in the care and management of the ill.

XI. *Wine as Vehicle for Medication*

||||||||||||||||||||||||||||||||||||||||||||||||||||||||||||||||||||||||||||||||||||||||||||||||||||||||||||||||||||||||||||||||||||||||||||||||||||||||||||||||||||||||||||||||

In ancient times, one of the important functions of wine was its use as a medium for the preparation and administration of medicinal agents. It also was utilized advantageously as a tonic and a regulator of the excretory organs.[1] Theophrastus[2] (4th century B.C.) described a multitude of medicinal plants decocted in wines. From Mnesitheus,[3] an Athenian physician of the same century, we have further substantiation of this reputed value as a vehicle. "In medicine it is most useful; it can be compounded with liquid drugs; it brings help to the wounded." Of the many classicists who emphasize wine as a vehicle for medication are Pliny,[4] his contemporary, Columella,[5] and Celsus.[6]

During the benighted era of Prohibition the use of alcohol in any form was frowned upon. The pharmacopoeial standards for Vinum Xericum, Vinum Portense, Vinum Album and Vinum Rubrum unfortunately were outlawed. Previously they had been described in the U.S. Pharmacopoeia, but because of the widespread emotional sentiment against alcohol pharmaceutical chemists were discouraged from using it and the pharmacists who were trained in that era remained unaware of its many virtues. The pendulum is now swinging back and wine is again brought into grace as the most useful and most economical solvent and vehicle for carrying the galenic agents. The wine types most frequently used in pharmaceutical chemistry are sherry and white port.

The white dry table wines are important as diuretics; and liquorous wines are employed to dissolve alterable drugs.[7] The advantages of wine over other alcoholic menstrua are several:

(*1*) the range of alcoholic concentration (7 to 21 per cent) is sufficient to keep relatively insoluble substances in solution;

(*2*) the greater solubility of many of the commonly used medications in mildly acid solutions;

(*3*) the pleasant, inexpensive flavoring provided by the aromatic organic esters of wine which obviate the need for costly foreign or synthetic extracts; and

(*4*) the buffering action attributable to the presence of natural salts of potassium and sodium in the form of tartrates and phosphates.

The excellent buffering action of wine undoubtedly is the reason for its popularity as a menstruum. The desiccated white wine extracts of U.S.P. Belladonna root so successful in the treatment of postencephalitic Parkinsonism have not been matched by any other preparation of like nature.[8] In these preparations, the superiority of the white wine as a solvent far surpasses that of any other hydroalcoholic combination. Neal and Dillenberg[9] failed to prepare so satisfactory a decoction when solvents other than white table wine were used, and Fabing and Zeligs[10] were equally unsuccessful in their search for a substitute.

Although today pharmaceutical chemists constantly utilize wine in compounding their preparations, statistical information on the extent of its use is unavailable. Manufacturers are notoriously reluctant to share their trade secrets. However, it is safe to say that wine, as a vehicle for medicaments, is as widely used as any other solvent. Wine "augments exceedingly the quality of the remedies with which it is mixed,"[11] and many an ardent teetotaler has found his favorite medication palatable because of the pleasant quality and mildly euphoric effect of the hidden wine it contains.

XII. *The Use of Wine in the Treatment of the Aged and the Convalescent*

||||||||||||||||||||||||||||||||||||||||||||||||||||||||||||||||||||||||||||||||||||||||||||||||||||||||||||||||||||||||||||||||||||||||||||||||||||||||||||||||||||||||||||||||||

Wine, the handmaiden for those myriad social and festive functions of a vigorous and youthful life, becomes a balm for the convalescent and "milk" for the aged. The autumnal years of life usually burdened by disenchantment and fatigue, and often lament, become bearable behind the aura of a glass of pleasant wine. Such thoughts have conditioned the attitude of those physicians, ancient and modern, who realize that the whole of existence is more than an addition of perfectly functioning organs. The allusions of Hippocrates, Galen and Celsus to the curative and restorative powers of wine have conditioned all, both lay and professional, who aspire to treat and alleviate the indispositions, real and imaginary, of man. Gardeton[1] has quaintly phrased his appraisal of the therapeutic value of wine in the following manner: "Wine is salutary for old persons and to feeble persons because it fortifies them greatly. In moderation it dissipates black melancholy and produces sleep." Gaubert[2] comments favorably on the "agreeable stimulation" of wine which he considers "a resource for aged persons whose digestion languishes," and a sovereign remedy "for persons exhausted from long illness."

Many persons of advanced age are accustomed to a daily alcoholic beverage. Unless they are acutely ill, it is a serious mistake to exclude alcohol from their regimen, "for the emotional factors thus disturbed might produce more harm than good."[3] Even those who have never used alcohol before "find advantage in their declining years in a more systematic use of wine or spirits."[4] Since early days the temperate use of wine has been prescribed in the care and treatment of the aged—not alone for its content of alcohol but for many other beneficial ingredients a good wine contains.

From France (where else?) comes a 19th-century testimonial in praise of its rejuvenative powers. When the Mayor of Beaune at the age of eighty sired his sixteenth child, the jubilant citizens attributed his vigor and virility to the generous quantity of burgundy he imbibed with his meals.[5] This tale of Gallic peasant origin is more than phantasy. There can be little doubt of the therapeutic value of wine in the alleviation of that indefinable indisposition characteristic of the involutionary period of life. Thewlis[6] says "many older persons suffer from indefinite symptoms such as sleeplessness, nervousness, numbness in the legs and arms, loss of appetite, indigestion, weakness, melancholia," fugitive pains at night, and a host of more occult complaints. Wine and its spirit, taken with food, will often suppress these myriad symptoms "because of the mild sedative effect of alcohol on the brain and spinal cord."

Haggard and Jellinek,[7] commenting upon the usefulness of alcohol in easing anxiety and pain, describe it as "unquestionably the safest of all sedatives." There is only one condition, they point out, in which "the utility of alcoholic beverages, in suitable moderation and low concentrations, is generally admitted and that is the bodily discomforts brought about by age." Taken with a little food at bedtime, wines—especially port—are highly recommended for insomnia. Anstie[8] observes that "one very important effect of the highly etherized wines is their power to produce tranquil and prolonged sleep in aged persons. Considering how simple a prescription this is, it is surprising how often its value is ignored by medical men." More recently Salter has stated that "for protracted use alcohol in moderation can serve as the old peoples' sedative."[9]

Hypertension, with its aggravating fears and anxieties, is often a penalty of advancing years. Alcohol is no panacea for the scourge, hypertension; but that it "does reduce pressure brought on by emotional factors seems beyond dispute. That it prolongs life and increases comfort is but a corollary of this fact."[10] For the hesitant heart, bothersomely irregular, alternately intermittent and frequently punctuated by breathlessness or a fleeting twinge, considerable comfort may be afforded by the discreet use of alcohol.[11]

As for those with normally advanced arteriosclerosis, the effects of small amounts of wine are unquestionably beneficial.[12] In the aged, loss of elasticity in arteries is due chiefly to the deposition of calcium in atheromatous plaques. Although the ingestion of wine does not reverse the process, it slows the rate of deposition of cholesterol, directly, and calcium, indirectly, in the intima of the blood vessels. The use of alcoholic beverages for this therapeutic purpose has been mentioned by Leary,[13] who considers the role of alcohol as a possible decholesterinizing agent. For the marasmus, frequently an accompaniment of senility, Loebenstein-Loebel[14] states that in his experience old and generous Madeira wines have proven to be excellent remedies for this preventable cachexia.

The food value of wine has been discussed in an earlier section where it was noted that there is yet much to be learned about those constituents of wine other than alcohol which contribute to its beneficial action upon the human body. We are still unfamiliar, for instance, with the role of amino acids in maintaining the soundness of the body. Some of these constituents may exert a restraining effect upon the involutionary processes. If so, the nutritive importance of wine for the aged is particularly significant. The ease with which it is metabolized is also an advantage to those who have passed the middle span of life. For them the desirable nourishment is that which can be absorbed, utilized and eliminated with the greatest dispatch. Those who suffer from hypochromic anemia gain an added benefit from the ingestion of alcohol in the form of wine. Its iron content, according to figures given by Bowes et al[15] indicate that it aids materially in combating the anemia so often found in this age group. By its carminative action, alcohol whets the appetite for nourishment in other forms. In reference to the lack of desire for food frequently present in later life, Einhorn[16] notes that "if we give people with anorexia small doses of an alcoholic beverage they are able to take their meals. Otherwise they would die."

Alcohol in itself is a proven means of aiding digestion and of enhancing caloric intake. "Whisky, brandy or wine," Thewlis[17] observes, "usually will improve the digestion if taken with meals." This is particularly important for the aged[18] who are more sensitive to vagaries of the digestive apparatus than are the young. Jackson stated: *"Cognac brandy* is like a carefully compounded medical prescription. Its principal component is alcohol, holding in solution certain synergists which enhance and complete its effectiveness."[19] The mild secretory stimulation that follows the ingestion of wine is beneficial to the generally lax and achlorhydric stomach of old age. Furthermore, experimentally in man and animals, alcohol implements other activities of the gastrointestinal tract: namely, it helps to solve the problem of adequate fluid intake; and by its tonic effect on the colon it facilitates the important gastrocolic reflexes which control the evacuatory functions.[20]

There is one salutary effect of wine that cannot be explained on the basis of objective, measurable data. It is what pharmacologists describe as the euphoric effect.[21] This connotes the glowing sensation of well-being which follows the temperate consumption of good wine. In that period of life too often marred by general indisposition, and the awareness of involution with its all-pervading sense of uselessness, what could be more desirable?

The widely-held opinion that "wine, prudently used, has naturally a strong and direct tendency to prolong life"[22] antedates modern medicine by many generations. One of the most celebrated stories of the therapeutic value of wine in longevity is told about an 18th-century Venetian nobleman, Cornaro, whose irregular life so ravaged his constitution that at the age of thirty-five he was given up by his physicians.[23] Barry[24] reports that on their advice—as a final, desperate measure—he reduced his diet "to a certain quantity of solids and fluids daily, which last consisted entirely of wine." By diminishing the quantity of each as he advanced in years, Cornaro lived to be 100.

Pearl[25] has discussed the problem of longevity and concludes that moderate drinking of alcoholic beverages does not significantly shorten life when compared with the life span of total abstainers. In a discussion of this problem in Billings'[26] symposium, it is stated that "a temperate use of light wines or diluted spirits, especially after the age of 55, is more conducive to longevity than is total abstinence." In a study of longevity in the wine regions of France, Fabre[27] found that, all factors being equal, the greatest longevity was among those who were accustomed to the moderate use of wine in their daily diet. Sorel[28] corroborates Fabre: "Statistics prove that the drinkers of water live a shorter time than wine drinkers and that it is in the wine regions that there are found fewer alcoholics and insane." In all discussions of the effects of wine upon longevity, the keynote of advice seems to be not excess or abstention, but moderation.

Whether wine be considered as sedative, medicine, food, digestive aid or a factor in longevity, it is indisputably a boon to the aged. "The argument in its favor when widely and prudently used, seems complete. It does us good and can do us no harm," says Farquharson.[29]

Convalescents, regardless of their years, share many of the recuperative and tonic needs of the aged. Therefore, the salutary effects of wine are equally valuable for those who are recovering from severe illnesses. Unless definitely contraindicated, Royer-Collard[30] prescribes wine in convalescence under any circumstances. Ollier[31] observes that the moderate use of wine produces excellent therapeutic results. It is also considered a "first rate tonic and an agent for rapid return to health."[32]

For illustrative purposes, Dale et al[33] cite the case of 70-year-old Sir Samuel Wilks. Upon his recovery from an attack of influenza, Sir Samuel carried about with him a small flask of wine. In the performance of his onerous duties, he derived great benefit by drinking from the flask whenever weakness and exhaustion overcame him. The authors consider his testimony valuable for here, they note, "we have evidence of an abstentious and scientific man making an observation upon himself."

Bégin[34] notes that wine taken in small quantities—one-half glass of claret either before or after meals—is "the surest and most hygienic way to restore the nutritional functions" as well as to reestablish "the vital forces." Producing as it does a flow of gastric juice, wine is valuable in conditions of depressed metabolism.[35] Pousson[36] further recommends it because of the part it plays in "increasing red corpuscles, the hemoglobin and the iron in the blood."

In recent years it has been discovered that as a tonic, vitamin B_1 suspended in wine is the best form in which the medication can be given. Greengard[37] cites experiments showing that in aqueous solutions, vitamin B_1 is precipitated as thiochrome, thereby rendering the vitamin medically ineffective. He reports that because of the greater stability of thiamin chloride in a mildly acid medium wine appears to be the most ideal and satisfactory menstruum for prescribing vitamin B_1.

It is clear, then, that physicians treating the aged and the convalescent have for generations been aware of the restorative powers of wine, which are due not only to its content of alcohol but also to other more beneficial ingredients. The carminative action of wine and the ease with which it is metabolized make it an important factor in nutrition. It also provides an increased intake of fluids which is highly desirable. For the gastrointestinal tract, wine performs several services: it stimulates the gastric secretion, improves the tone of the colon, and facilitates the evacuatory functions. Wine is considered by many to be the safest of all sedatives and is used for this effect in alleviating the vague disturbances characteristic of the involutionary cycle. Prudent quantities of wine are helpful in reducing the emotional pressure which aggravates hypertension, in relieving the discomfort of heart conditions associated with advanced age, and in delaying the progress of arteriosclerosis. The opinion is held widely both here and abroad that wine may be conducive to longevity. There is no doubt that taken with discretion it adds greatly to the pleasures of the table, to physical comfort, and to mental serenity in the aged. The generalized vasodilatation, the increased flow of blood to the skin, and the mild euphoria wine produces are as necessary as they are gratifying to both the aged and the convalescent.

XIII. *The Elixir of the Grape*

||||||||||||||||||||||||||||||||||||||||||||||||||||||||||||||||||||||||||||||||||||||||||||||||||||||||||||||||||||||||||||||||||||||||||||||||||||||

The elixir of the grape, sweet wine, curiously has been the pride of master wine makers from ancient times, and basically reflects the care and attention that must accompany the production of such nectar. Wherever in the world sweet wines are made, the appropriate well-ripened grapes are carefully pressed and processed, the expressed juice is meticulously tended, and the fermentation arrested at that point where the quantity of alcohol and residual sugar are such that the best bloom of the vintage will be preserved in the finished wine. The end result is a sweet and luscious elixir called, variously, sweet wine, dessert wine, apéritif, and cordial wine. The short fermentation period of sweet wines results in a lesser quantity of extractive substances, fewer by-products of fermentation, and greater quantities of residual sugar than is found in the table wines. Alcohol, in the form of brandy, is selectively added to arrest fermentation of the specific type of grape at that point at which the desired degree of sweetness is attained for the characteristic variety of wine desired. Furthermore, the quantity of acids present in the wine following fermentation is less than the potential quantity naturally present in the fully ripened grapes, thus accounting for the relative flatness of sweet wines when compared with table wines. The addition of brandy to sweet wines, although it limits the amount and character of the fruit acids in the finished product, enhances its alcohol content and adds the restorative power of ethyl alcohol and its esters to the medicinal virtues of the organic compounds found in the basic wine.

Due to differences in the mode of production and blending, dessert wines differ from table wines in several ways: they contain fewer extractive substances and by-products of fermentation, more residual sweetness, and markedly different proportions of acids, aldehydes and esters of potential biologic value. The alcohol of the brandy which is added to sweet wines causes the tartrates to precipitate more readily, promotes the extraction of substances from the wooden casks in which the wine is stored, and enhances the solubility and miscibility of certain organic substances. The natural aging of sweet wines at reduced temperatures for long periods of time or the accelerated aging in moderately warm cellars may selectively intensify these effects. One of the factors responsible for the specific flavor of dessert wines, namely the sweetness and relative blandness attributed to the lowered content of fixed acid, is traceable in part to the variety of grapes used, the effect of the climate upon their maturation, the period at which fermentation was interrupted, and the temperature at which maturation was effected. The addition of brandy reduces the acidity of the finished wine and this influences its quality; therefore, the higher the total fixed acid content of the grape varieties used in the production of sweet wines the greater the possibility of capturing that special acid and ester balance which renders certain of these wines unique.

There are various types of sweet wines; the best known are Port and Sherry. As far as we know, Port was the first wine in which the principle of arrested fermentation was used, and it was the forerunner of all dessert wines. For the excellence of Port, its culture and wide popularity, we are indebted to the English, who consider it to be essentially the wine of philosophic contemplation. Saintsbury has said

that "it strengthens while it gladdens as no other wine can
do; and there is something about it which must have been
created in pre-established harmony with the best English
character."[1] Port demands and produces a solemn mood—
scholarly but not pedantic—in which the amateur soars
through problems of metaphysics with ease and Gordian
intricacies with mastery. The ultimate question—whether
the external world exists or not—is less pertinent than that
Port wine is extremely good. Vintage port, weighted though
it may be with the memories of great conversationalists, is
never ordinary; as the decanter is passed among the vo-
taries, their discourses glow with a rich and companionate
solemnity. Port is at its best in an atmosphere of serious
and leisurely contemplation, an atmosphere that can scarcely
be penetrated by the currently superficial spirit with its
craze for speed and its contempt for the naturally slow
maturation of men and ideas.[2] It is easily understandable
that a wine so big, so robust, so warm and glowing would
find its best use in a cold bleak climate where its sweetness
gives energy while its alcohol warms the heart and stimulates the mind.

"Port stands pre-eminent amongst wines as a full, rich
and strength-giving stimulant."[3] It has long been used as
a stomachic to combat the anorexia of debilitating diseases,
protracted fevers,[4] various infections,[5] and tuberculosis.[6]
It has also been advised as a tonic and an aid to digestion
in the enfeebled.[7] It is especially valuable when given to the
aged,[8] for whom "the fine volatile ethers which develop in
well-kept old bottled Port and Sherry have an extraordinary
influence in heightening the stimulant and tonic effect of
alcohol."[9] To combat insomnia, that troublesome torment,
no remedy is more sovereign than a glass of brilliant Port
taken before retiring.[10] Brande said: "Good Port Wine,
duly kept, is, when taken in moderation, one of the most
wholesome of vinous liquors. It strengthens the muscular
system, assists the digestive powers, accelerates the circu-

lation, exhilarates the spirits, and sharpens the mental energies."[11]

In a Treatise on Fever, published in Edinburgh in 1785, Dr. Caleb Dickinson concludes: "Wine may, perhaps, in a great measure, supercede many other stimulants in the cure of fever; and it has this great advantage over all others, of being generally agreeable to the palate . . . Of all the wines that are presented to us, I think red Port answers the purpose as well as any other."[12]

In the 19th century, vast quantities of Port were consumed in England, but toward the end of this period it became "abused with indiscriminate vehemence"[13] for its imputed gout-producing properties. In regard to the etiology of gout, it is apparent to modern investigators that it is less a matter of the consumption of Port wine, and more a problem of the internal environment and the manner in which a person metabolizes purines, conditioned somewhat by the region in which a person lives and other external environmental features of his living.

Sherry, another elixir, similar in many respects to Port, differs markedly in that other varieties of grapes are used; the wine is subjected to double fermentation and blended in order to produce wines of varying degrees of dryness and sweetness, and ultimately given a quantity of brandy for purposes of stabilization and preservation. It is the medicinal wine *par excellence* since both dry and sweet varieties can be used as tonics, stomachics, and sedatives. The dry variety is in great demand as a universal vehicle for medicinal agents. "Sherry wine is more often used as a vehicle for medicinal ingredients than any other wine, . . . because of its general availability, its high alcohol content, its uniformity, and stability. At present it is the only wine specified in the National Formulary."[14]

"Now as to the uses of sherry," says Dr. Druitt,[15] "good old sherry is a most valuable cordial and stomachic, and has marvelous uses for stimulating a feeble heart and making a refractory stomach do its work. And if patients or physicians desire to take or prescribe sherry, let me say with that great animal, Martin Luther, *Pecca fortiter,* do the thing handsomely; keep a reserve of fine old sherry for infirmity, and use it thankfully."

Dr. Anstie heralded the "highly ethereal wines" as distinctively indicated for the cardiac exhaustion accompanying the long-continued fevers common in his day. He prescribed fine old sherry, 6 to 12 ounces per day, in divided doses given at one-half hour intervals and remarked: "it is surprising how rapidly this treatment at the same time restores strength and regularity to the heart's action, and calms the nervous system, so as to allow of sweet and restorative sleep." He was "convinced that the influence of such a liquor is something entirely distinct from that of its mere alcohol."[16]

A unique use of sherry wine was also recorded by Anstie, who stated that "Very acute neuralgia may sometimes appear to demand the use of alcohol; and the power of alcoholic stimulants, especially of good sherry, to relieve such pain is an unquestionable fact."[17]

A more modern eulogy of sherry is that of Warner Allen, who says: "It has something in it of the tonic quality of sea air, for it instantly stimulates the sensory nerves and awakens interest in life."[18]

Among other elixirs of the grape may be mentioned Madeira wine, which is in many respects similar to sherry excepting that it has been subjected to baking at elevated temperatures and subsequently given an addition of brandy. The Madeira wines are sweet and are used as tonics, stomachics and restoratives. Madeira "abounds in the truest vinous elements; it is a most potent stimulant to the nerves."[19] "It is a singular circumstance, that *Madeira wine* should afford no tartar as other wines do, and must therefore consequently contain a quantity of fixed alkali, in an uncombined state: on this account most probably it is, that invalids, . . . with depraved appetites, and weak stomachs disposed to acidity, find it to agree with them better than other wines."[20]

Unfortunately there have been no champions of the wines of Madeira equal in eloquence to those in praise of Port and Sherry. On the other hand, there have been some lay proponents of Tokay Essence who have said many extravagant things concerning this remarkable wine. One such is mentioned by Berry: "Someone described it as the wine that would take the screws out of a coffin lid."[21] To an Englishman of Mr. Berry's zeal, the juice of the grape in some form was a worthy panacea for all ills. "A Tokay Essence with a mere 3 per cent. of alcohol will produce the most amazing restorative effects and bring back the sick from the very edge of the grave. An ordinary Tokay wine with 15 per cent. of alcohol is comparatively powerless."[22]

In a letter to Dr. Buchan concerning the medical virtues of wine, an extensive discussion concerns the marvelous curative effects upon the gastrointestinal tract of a generous cordial wine referred to as Tokay de Espagna, which was heralded as a remedy for the nervous and weak, those afflicted with bilious indigestion, depressed spirits, melancholia, lack of appetite, diarrhea, obstruction of the urinary passages, and malarial fever.[23] The Tokay de Espagna may have been the Spanish muscatelle called *Lagrima,* a wine made of the virgin juice of Malaga grapes which had been allowed to hang in the open air and whose natural juice was caught as it trickled down without any sort of pressure from the very ripe bunches of grapes.

The Muscatels are among the sweetest of the elixirs of the grape, and as their quantities of fixed acids are increased, they become even more excellent in quality. They are highly aromatic because the distinctive bloom which gives character to the grape is carried over into the wine, imparting to it a rich and luscious flavor. Wines made from the muscat grapes are of ancient origin and at some time

or other they have been produced in practically every viti-
cultural district of the world. The wine Est! Est!! Est!!!
made famous by the Bishop of Fulda, is a product of this
grape, as are many Italian vermouths, or medicated wines,
which are the modern day counterpart and remnants of
those famous Theriacs of the Middle Ages.

There are many other vinous elixirs which have been
used to stimulate the appetite of the convalescent and bring
cheer to those racked by illness. Among them may be mentioned the natural sweet French Sauternes, the German
Trockenbeeren ausleses and spätleses; the Italian Marsalas,
the Malmseys, Malvoisies, and Malagas which belong to
the broad group of Madeiras—all of which have enjoyed
special attention and popularity.

The elixirs of the grape are precious ammunition and
offer a balm to the therapeutist whose genius can call upon
them to brighten a dulled psyche, to cajole a wayward appetite, to pacify an overwrought bowel, to banish the foes of
Hypnos, and to bring hope reminiscent of youth to the
autumnal years of those enfeebled by the execrations of
old age.

References

I. The Chemistry of Wine

General:

Amerine, M. A., and M. A. Joslyn: *Table Wines,* Berkeley, University of California Press, 1951.

Cruess, W. V.: *The Principles and Practice of Wine Making,* New York, Avi Publishing Co., Inc., 1947.

Genevois, L., et J. Ribéreau-Gayon: *Le Vin,* Paris, Hermann et Cie., 1947.

Joslyn, M. A., and M. A. Amerine: *Commercial Production of Brandies* (Bulletin ⚹652), Berkeley, University of California Press, 1941.

Mulder, G. J.: *The Chemistry of Wine,* London, John Churchill, 1857.

Reich, P.: *Wein-Kompendium für den Arzt,* Stuttgart, Wissenschaftliche Verlagsgesellschaft, M. b. H., 1950.

Ribéreau-Gayon, J., et E. Peynaud: *Analyse et Contrôle des Vins,* Paris et Liège, Librairie Polytechnique, Ch. Béranger, 1951.

Valaer, P.: *Wines of the World,* New York, Abelard Press, Inc., 1950.

II. The Physiologic Effects of Wine

General:

Burbridge, T. N., and C. H. Hine: *J. Pharmacol. Exper. Therap.,* **103**:338 (1951).

Reich, Philipp: *Wein-Kompendium für den Arzt,* Stuttgart, Wissenschaftliche Verlagsgesellschaft, M. b. H., 1950.

Specific:

1. Dragstedt, C. A., et al.: *Proc. Soc. Exper. Biol. & Med.,* **43**:26 (1940).
2. Mellanby, E.: Medical Research Council. (Special Report ⚹31) 1919.

3. Carpenter, Thorne M.: *Quart. J. Alcohol,* 1:201–226 (1940).
4. Mitchell, H. H., and E. G. Curzon: *Quart. J. Alcohol,* 1:228–245 (1940).
5. Widmark, E. M. P.: *Biochem. Zschr.,* 265:237 (1933).
6. Levick, G. M.: *Practitioner,* 128:191 (1932).
7. Neymark, M., and E. M. P. Widmark: *Scand. Arch. Physiol.,* 73:260 (1936).
8. Newman, H. W., and W. C. Cutting: *J. Pharmacol. & Exper. Therap.,* 54:371–377 (1935).
9. Widmark, E. M. P.: *Biochem. Zschr.,* 259:285 (1933).
10. Lilienfeld-Toailles, Pavel F.: *Concours méd.,* 62:967 (1940).
11. Mitchell and Curzon: *Op. cit.*
12. *Ibid.*
13. Völtz, W., and J. Pächtner: *Biochem. Zschr.,* 42:73 (1913).
14. Irvin, D. L., A. Durra, and F. R. Goetzl: *Am. J. Digest. Dis.,* 20:17 (1953).
15. Gardner, J.: personal communication to the author of unpublished data.

III. Wine as a Food

1. Cuvier, F.: *Le Vin,* Paris Thèse ♯200, 1932.
2. Tant, E.: (Abst.) *Off. Internat. du Vin Bul.,* 23:91–97 (1950).
3. Maria Rosa: (Résumé) *Off. Internat. du Vin Bul.,* 17–18:102 (1944).
4. Llagnet: *J. de méd. de Bordeaux,* 108:1065 (1931).
5. Ray, Georges: *Vins de France,* Paris, University Press, 1946 (p. 75).
6. *Hippocrates:* Cambridge, Harvard University Press, 1939.
7. *Athenaeus:* New York, G. P. Putnam's Sons, 1927–1941.
8. *Galen:* New York, G. P. Putnam's Sons, 1928.
9. Celsus: *De Medicina,* Cambridge, Harvard University Press, 1935.
10. Guyot, J.: *Culture de la Vigne et Vinification,* Paris, Librairie Agricole de la Maison Rustique, 1861 (p. 377).
11. Stoll, H. F.: *Wine-Wise,* San Francisco, Crocker, 1933 (p. 10).

12. Loeper, M.: "Conference on the Cellular Activity of Wine," *Off. Internat. du Vin Bul.,* **10**:2 (1937).

13. Lozano, E. H.: *Rev. Vin. y de Indust. Anexas,* **10**:17 (1939).

14. Bunker, H. J.: *Nutritive Value of Yeast, Beer, Wines and Spirits,* (Chemical Industries, No. 16) 1947 (pp. 203–205).

15. Tant: *Op. cit.*

16. Dontas, S.: *Off. Internat. du Vin Bul.,* **7**:2 (1934).

17. Jager, J.: *Médecine,* **19**:990 (1938).

18. *Encyclopedia Britannica,* 13th ed., 1926 (p. 1037).

19. Koren, John: *Alcohol and Society,* New York, Henry Holt & Co., Inc., 1916 (p. 161).

20. Proust, L.: *Arch. du Droit Méd. et de l'Hyg.,* p. 9 (March 1, 1932).

21. Bridges, M. A.: *Dietetics for the Clinician,* Philadelphia, Lea & Febiger, 1941 (p. 862).

22. Duhamel, Georges: (quoted by R. J. Weissenbach) *Off. Internat. du Vin Bul.,* **22**:46 (1949).

23. Biester, Alice, M. W. Wood, and C. S. Wahlin: *Am. J. Physiol.,* **73**:387–396 (1925).

24. Gettler, A. O.: *J. Am. Chem. Soc.,* **54**:76 (1932).

25. Parisi, E., M. Sacchetti, and C. Bruini: *Ann. Chim. appl. Roma,* **22**:616–620 (1932).

26. Amerine, M. A., and M. A. Joslyn: *Commercial Production of Dessert Wines,* (University of California Agricultural Experimental Station Bulletin ⚡651) Berkeley, 1941.

27. Gottschalk, A.: *Biochem. J.,* **40**:621–626 (1946).

28. Engler, G. A.: *Wines and Vines* (November 1941).

29. Connor, C. L.: *J.A.M.A.,* **112**:387–390 (1939).

30. Chaikoff, I. L., C. L. Connor, and G. R. Biskind: *Am. J. Path.,* **14**:101–110 (1938).

31. Tappeiner, H.: *Zschr. Biol.,* **16**:497 (1880).

32. Brandl, J.: *Zschr. Biol.,* **29**:277 (1892).

33. von Scanzoni, F.: *Zschr. Biol.,* **33**:462 (1896).

34. Higgins, H. L.: *Am. J. Physiol.,* **41**:258–265 (1916).

35. Edkins, N.: *J. Physiol.,* **65**:381–384 (1928).

36. Edkins, N., and M. M. Murray: *J. Physiol.,* **66**:102–108 (1928); and **71**:403–411 (1931).

37. Neumann, R. O.: *München. med. Wchnschr.,* **48**:1126 (1901).

38. Atwater, W. O., and F. G. Benedict: *Mem. Nat. Acad. Sc.,* **8**:235–297 (1902).
39. Dougnac, F.: *Le Vin, aux Points de Vue Physico-chimique, Physiologique, Hygiénique, Thérapeutique.* Delmas, Chapon, Gounouilhou, 1935 (p. 83).
40. Fishbein, W., J. K. Calvin, and J. Heumann: *Arch. Pediat.,* **55**:42–45 (1938).
41. Randoin, Lucie: *Bull. Soc. scient. d'hyg. aliment.,* **16**:466 (1928).
42. Morgan, A. F., H. L. Nobles, A. Wiens, G. L. Marsh, and A. J. Winkler: *Food Research,* **4**:217–229 (1939).
43. Underwood, E. J.: *Nutrition Abstr. & Rev.,* **9**:515–534 (1940).
44. Amerine, M. A., and M. A. Joslyn: *Commercial Production of Table Wines* (University of California Agricultural Experimental Station Bulletin #639) 1940 (pp. 18–22).
45. Amerine, M. A., and T. T. Kishaba: *Proc. Am. Soc. Enol.,* **3**:77–86 (1952).
46. Eiler, J. J., M. Stockholm, and T. L. Althausen: *J. Biol. Chem.,* **134**:283–291 (1940).
47. a) Elvehjem, C. A., H. Steenbock, and E. B. Hart: *J. Biol. Chem.,* **83**:21–25 (1929).
    b) Voegtlin, C., J. M. Johnson, and S. M. Rosenthal: *Pub. Health Rep.,* **46**:2234–2253 (1931).
48. Saywell, L. G., and B. B. Cunningham: *Indust. & Engin. Chem.,* (anal. edition), **9**:67–69 (1937).
49. Dougnac: *Op. cit.* (pp. 77–81).
50. Atwater, W. O., and F. G. Benedict: *Mem. Nat. Acad. Sc.,* **8**:231 (1902).
51. Mitchell, H. H.: *J. Nutrition,* **10**:311 (1935).
52. Albertoni and Rossi: *Mém. de l'Acad. Royale des Sc. de l'Inst. de Biol. de Bologne;* quoted by Dougnac: *Op. cit.* (p. 80).
53. Richter, Curt P.: *Quart. J. Alcohol,* **1**:650–662 (1941).
54. Eylaud and R. Marcard: *Off. Internat. du Vin Bul.,* **6**:93 (1933).
55. Cuvier: *Op. cit.*
56. Foveau de Courmelles: *Hyg. Soc.,* p. 497 (July, 1935).
57. Clauera: (Abstract) *Off. Internat. du Vin Bul.,* **23**:103 (1950).

58. Weissenbach, R. J.: *Off. Internat. du Vin Bul.*, **22**:46 (1929).
59. Jager: *Op. cit.*
60. Christie, W. F.: *Practitioner*, **129**:721–729 (1932).
61. Weissenbach: *Op. cit.*

IV. The Action of Wine upon the Digestive Organs and its Use in Diseases of the Gastrointestinal System

1. Bullein, William: *Government of Health*, 1595 (Quoted by Gustafson, Axel) *Foundation of Death*, Boston, Ginn & Company, 1885.
2. Marescalchi, A.: *L'Italia Vinicola ed Agraria*, **28**:313–314 (1938).
3. Trullols Mateu, S.: *Sabor de España*, Igualada, 1947 (p. 25).
4. Mallory, W. J.: *M. Rec.*, **100**:275 (1921).
5. Pachon, V. (Quoted by Delaunay, H., and G. Portmann): *Off. Internat. du Vin Bul.*, **3**:55 (1930).
6. Loeper, Maurice, and J. Alquier: *Progr. méd., Paris*, **44**:1725–1730 (1929).
7. Billings, J. S., et al.: *Physiological Aspects of the Liquor Problem*, New York, Houghton Mifflin Co., 1903 (p. 148).
8. Roberts, Sir William: *Collected Contributions on Digestion and Diet*, London, Smith, Elder, 1897 (p. 134).
9. Buchner; quoted by Billings: *Op. cit.* (p. 188).
10. Billings: *Op. cit.* (pp. 188–189).
11. *Ibid.* (p. 195).
12. Carlson, A. J.: *Control of Hunger in Health and Disease*, Chicago, University of Chicago Press, 1916.
13. Roberts, Sir William: *Op. cit.*
14. Beaurepaire, L. B.: *Dissertation sur le Vin.* Paris Thèse ✕155, 1831.
15. Loeper and Alquier: *Op. cit.*
16. Chittenden, R. H., L. B. Mendel, and H. C. Jackson: *J. Physiol.*, **1**:164 (1898).
17. Winsor, A. L., and E. I. Strongin: *Exper. Psychol.*, **16**:589–597 (1933).

18. Beazell, J. M., and A. C. Ivy: *Quart. J. Alcohol,* **1**:45–73 (1940).
19. Linde, P: *Arch. f. exper. Path. u. Pharmakol.,* **167**:285–291 (1932).
20. Abels, J. C.: *Proc. Soc. Exper. Biol. & Med.,* **34**:346–351 (1936).
21. Vollenbruck, H.: *Arch. f. exper. Path. u. Pharmakol.,* **187**:731 (1937).
22. Friedmann, F. E., W. G. Motel, and H. J. Necheles: *J. Lab. & Clin. Med.,* **23**:1007 (1938).
23. Webb, W. W., R. B. Mullenix, and C. A. Dragstedt: *Proc. Soc. Exper. Biol. & Med.,* **29**:895–897 (1932).
24. Kast, L.: *Arch. Verdau. Kr.,* **12**:487 (1906).
25. Carlson: *Op. cit.* (p. 271).
26. Saito, S.: *Virchow's Arch.,* **185**:524 (1906).
27. Babkin, B. P.: *Die aussere Sekretien der Verdauungsdrusen,* Berlin, Julius Springer, 1928.
28. Barlow, O. W.: *J. Pharmacol. & Exper. Therap.,* **56**:117–146 (1936).
29. Dragstedt, C. A., J. S. Gray, A. H. Lawton, and M. Ramirez de Arellano: *Proc. Soc. Exper. Biol. & Med.,* **43**:26–28 (1940).
30. Barlow: *Op. cit.*
31. Mareschalchi: *Op. cit.*
32. Weissenbach, R. J., and Faroy: *Bull. Médecins Amis des Vins de France, IV Congrès,* **6**:88 (1937).
33. Kast, L.: *Biochem. Zbl.,* **5**:483 (1906).
34. Lönnquist, B.: *Scand. Arch. Physiol.,* **18**:241 (1906).
35. Babkin: *Op. cit.*
36. Krueger, L., and F. C. MacIntosh: *Am. J. Digest. Dis.,* **4**:104–107 (1937).
37. Haneborg, A.: *The Effect of Alcohol on Digestion in the Stomach,* Christiania, Grondahl & Son, 1921.
38. Ogden, Eric: personal communication to the author.
39. Scott, C. C., W. W. Scott, and A. B. Luckhardt: *Am. J. Physiol.,* **123**:248–255 (1938).
40. Beaurepaire: *Op. cit.*
41. Beckers, René: *Wines and Vines,* **21**(2), (1940).

42. Ferrannini, Andrea: *Riforma med.,* **45**:1730–1731 (1929).
43. Adler, H. F., J. M. Beazell, A. J. Atkinson, and A. C. Ivy: *Quart. J. Alcohol,* **1**:638–643 (1941).
44. Kuwschinski, P.: Diss. St. Petersburg, 532, 1888; quoted by Gizelt, A.: *Pflüger's Arch. f. d. ges. Physiol.,* **111**:620 (1906).
45. Gizelt, A.: *Pflüger's Arch. f. d. ges. Physiol.,* **111**:620 (1906).
46. Fleig, C.: *Compt. rend. Soc. de biol.,* **55**:1279 (1903).
47. Brooks, F. P., and J. E. Thomas: *Gastroenterology,* **23**:36 (1953).
48. Dreiling, D. A., A. Richman, and N. F. Fradkin: *Gastroenterology,* **20**:636 (1952).
49. Loeper, M., L. Michaux, and S. de Sèze: *Société Médicale des Hôpitaux de Paris* (Bull. et Mém.), **53**:1212 (1929).
50. Dougnac: *Op. cit.* (p. 93).
51. Loeper, M., L. Michaux, and S. de Sèze: *Op. cit.*
52. *Ibid.*
53. Valin et Laborde: *Bull. Acad. nat. méd.,* (October 12–19, 1897).
54. Mauriac, E.: *Défense du Vin au Triple Point de Vue Économique, Hygiénique, et Thérapeutique,* 10ᵉ Int. Congrès d'Hygiène et de Démographie, Paris, 1900.
55. Fiessinger, C.: *Vingt Régimes Alimentaires en Clientèle,* Paris, 1930 (quoted by Dougnac: *Op. cit.* p. 97).
56. Weissenbach and Faroy: *Op. cit.*

V. The Action of Wine upon the Respiratory System

1. Billings, J. S., et al.: *Physiological Aspects of the Liquor Problem,* Vol. 2, New York, Houghton Mifflin Co., 1903 (p. 106).
2. Wendelstadt; quoted by Billings: *Op. cit.* (p. 107).
3. LeBreton, E.: *Compt. rend. Soc. de biol.,* **117**:704 (1934).
4. Southgate, H. W., and G. Carter: *Brit. M. J.,* **1**:463 (1926).
5. Harger, R. N., E. B. Lamb, and H. R. Hulpieu: *J. A. M. A.,* **110**:779–785 (1938).
6. Haggard, H. W., and L. A. Greenberg: *J. Pharmocol. & Exper. Therap.,* **52**:164–165 (1934).

7. a) Hunter, F. T., and S. G. Mudd: *Boston Med. Surg. J.,* **190**:971 (1924).

   b) Robinson, L. J., and S. Selesnick: *J. A. M. A.,* **105**:1734–1738 (1935).

   c) McFarland, R. A., and A. L. Barach: *Am. J. M. Sc.,* **192**:186–198 (1936).

8. Newman, H. W., and J. Card: *J. A. M. A.,* **106**:595–596 (1936).

9. Brooks, C.: *J. A. M. A.,* **55**:372 (1910).

10. Hyatt, E. G.: *J. Lab. & Clin. Med.,* **5**:56 (1919).

11. Grubbs, R. C., and F. A. Hitchcock: *J. Nutrition,* **15**:229–244 (1938).

12. Celsus: *De Medicina,* Cambridge, Harvard University Press, 1935.

13. Graham, William: *The Art of Making Wines,* London, J. Williams, 1750.

14. Martinet, Alfred: *Thérapeutique Clinique,* Vol. 2, Paris, Masson et Cie, 1921.

15. Spilsbury, E. A.: *Lancet,* **7**:35 (1939).

16. Cruchet, R.: *J. de méd. de Bordeaux,* **110**:825 (1933).

17. Jager, J.: *La Valeur Alimentaire et Thérapeutique du Vin,* Paris Thèse ※550, 1938.

18. Young, R. A., and G. E. Beaumont; quoted by Price, F. W.: *Textbook of the Practice of Medicine,* London, Oxford University Press, 1946.

19. Jager, J.: *Médecine,* **19**:992 (1938).

VI. The Action of Wine upon the Cardio-vascular System

1. Arnald of Villanova: *The Earliest Printed Book on Wine* (?1235–1311), translation and introduction by Henry Sigerist; New York, Henry Schuman, Inc., 1943 (p. 35).

2. Moerchen: *Off. Internat. du Vin Bul.,* **3**:51 (1930).

3. Pardee, Harold E. B.; quoted by Harlow Brooks: *Med. J. & Rec.,* **127**:204 (1928).

4. Pons, C., and Broeckaert: *Belg. Méd.,* **16**:231–234 (1909).

5. a) Charcot, J. M., et al.: *Traité de Médecine,* Paris, Masson et Cie., 1899–1905 (Vol. 8, p. 224).
   b) Llagnet. *J. de méd. de Bordeaux,* 108 (1931).
   c) Guillermin, R.: quoted from *Traité de Médecine de Sergent,* 28:415, June 8, 1939.
6. Dontas, S.: *Off. Internat. du Vin Bul.,* 7:2 (1934).
7. Dieulafoy, G.: *A Textbook of Medicine,* Vol. 1, New York, Appleton, 1912 (p. 435).
8. Fitch, William; quoted by C. A. Rosewater: *J. M. Soc. New Jersey,* 16:276 (1919).
9. Heberden, William: *Med. Tr. Roy. Coll. Phys.,* 2:59 (1768).
10. Brooks, Harlow: *Med. J. & Rec.,* 127:201 (1928).
11. Clark, A. J.: *Applied Pharmacology,* London, J. & A. Churchill, 1929.
12. Stockton, C. G.: *M. Rec.,* 100:278 (1921).
13. Bishop, L. F.: *M. Rec.,* 100:280 (1921).
14. a) Starling, E. H.: *The Action of Alcohol on Man,* New York, Longmans, Green & Co., Inc., 1923 (pp. 137–138).
    b) Hare, H. A.: *A Textbook of Practical Therapeutics,* Philadelphia, Lea & Febiger, 1925.
    c) Hunt, W. R.: *Mississippi Doctor,* 16:13 (1939).
15. Cook, E. N., and G. E. Brown: *Proc. Mayo Clin.,* 7:449 (1932).
16. Parkes, E. A., and C. Wollowicz: *Proc. Roy. Soc. Med.,* London, 19:74 (1870).
17. Loeb, O.: *Arch. f. exp. Path. u. Pharmakol.,* 52:459 (1905).
18. Bachem, C.: *Arch. internat. de pharmacodyn.,* 14:437 (1905).
19. Dixon, W. E.: *J. Physiol.,* 35:346 (1906–1907).
20. Sulzer, R., and R. K. Cannan: *Heart Bull.,* 11:146–150 (1924).
21. Kootataladse, T. G.: *Russ. Physiol. J.,* 2:1 (1919).
22. Cabot, R. L.: *J. A. M. A.,* 43:774 (1904).
23. Lieb, C. C.: *J. A. M. A.,* 64:898 (1915).
24. Abel, J.; quoted by Billings: *Op. cit.* (Vol. 2, p. 91).
25. McDowell, R. J. S.: *J. Pharmacol. & Exper. Therap.,* 25:289–295 (1925).
26. Master, A. M., S. Dack, and H. L. Jaffe: *J. A. M. A.,* 109:546–549 (1937).
27. Eberhard, T. P.: *Arch. Path.,* 21:616–627 (1936).

28. Wilder, R. M.; quoted by Haven Emerson: *Alcohol and Man,* New York, The Macmillan Co., 1939 (p. 154).

VII. The Action of Wine upon the Kidneys and its Use in Renal Disease

1. Bright, Richard: *Reports of Medical Cases,* (Vol. 1, p. 29), London, Longmans, Green & Co., Inc., 1827.
2. Dickinson: *Treatise on Albuminuria,* New York, 1881, page 274; quoted by A. M. Fishberg: *Hypertension and Nephritis,* 4th Ed. (p. 609), Philadelphia, Lea & Febiger, 1939.
3. Fahr, T.: *Handbuch der speziellen pathologischen Anatomie und Histologie* (editors: Henke, F., and Lubarsch, O.) Vol. 7, Berlin, J. Springer, 1925 (p. 426).
4. Fishberg, A. M.: *Hypertension and Nephritis,* 4th Ed., Philadelphia, Lea & Febiger, 1939 (pp. 609–610).
5. Friedenwald, J.: *J. A. M. A.,* 45:781–783 (1905).
6. MacNider, W. de B.: *J. Pharmacol. & Exper. Therap.,* 26:100 (1925).
7. Bruger, M., S. A. Localio, and N. W. Guthrie: *J. A. M. A.,* 112:1782 (1939).
8. Wegelin, C.: *Schweiz. med. Wchnschr.,* 61:1181 (1931).
9. Cohnheim, J., and R. Marchand; quoted in editorial, *J. A. M. A.,* 98:2213 (1932).
10. Ziegler, L. H., and H. C. Horner: *New York State J. Med.,* 35:921 (1935).
11. Widmark, E. M. P.: *Scand. Arch. Physiol.,* 33:85 (1916).
12. Miles, W. R.: *J. Pharmacol. & Exper. Therap.,* 20:316 (1923).
13. Haggard, H. W., and L. A. Greenberg: *J. Pharmacol. & Exper. Therap.,* 52:164–165 (1934).
14. a) Labbé, Marcel: *Régimes Alimentaires,* Paris, Baillière, 1917.
    b) Dougnac, F.: *Le Vin aux Points de Vue Physio-Chimique, Physiologique, Hygiénique, Thérapeutique,* Delmas, Chapon, Gounouilhou, 1935 (p. 107).
    c) Weissenbach, R. J.: *Hôpital,* 24:80 (1936).
15. Bruger, Localio, and Guthrie: *Op. cit.*

16. John, M.: *Ztschr. f. exper. Path. u. Therap.,* **5**:579 (1909).

17. Bastedo, W. A.: *Materia Medica, Pharmacology and Therapeutics,* 3rd Ed., Philadelphia, W. B. Saunders Co., 1932, (p. 393).

18. Carles, P.: *J. de méd. de Bordeaux,* p. 597 (17 Sept., 1911); quoted by Dougnac: *Op. cit.* (p. 108).

19. Vincent, A. J. B.: *De Certains Réactions du Rein à Nos Vins Blancs Régionaux,* Paris Thèse ⚹38, 1931 (p. 27).

20. Dougnac: *Op. cit.* (p. 107).

21. Weissenbach: *Op. cit.*

22. Mrak, E. M., and J. H. Fessler: *Ztschr. f. Untersuch. d. Lebensmitt.,* **72**:461 (1936).

23. Saywell, L. G.: *J. Nutrition,* **5**:103 (1932).

24. Clouse, R. C.: *J. Nutrition,* **9**:593 (1935).

25. Labbé: *Op. cit.*

26. Manquat, A.: *Traité élémentaire de Thérapeutique,* Vol. 2, Paris, Baillière, 1918 (p. 450).

27. Mosenthal, H. O.: *Variations in Blood Pressure and Nephritis,* Oxford Monographs, vii. New York, Oxford University Press, 1929.

28. Van Noorden, C.; quoted by F. Vogelius: *Acta med. Scandinav.* (supp.), **7**:309 (1924).

29. Fishberg: *Op. cit.*

30. Dougnac: *Op. cit.,* (p. 273).

31. Bruger, M.: *Quart. J. Alcohol,* **1**:85–94 (1940).

VIII. The Action of Wine upon the Neuromuscular System

1. Billings, J. S., et al.: *Physiological Aspects of the Liquor Problem,* New York, Houghton Mifflin Co., 1903 (p. 117).

2. Kraepelin; quoted by Billings: *Op. cit.* (p. 142).

3. Mitscherlich and Schmiedeberg; quoted by Billings: *Op. cit.* (p. 120).

4. Moerchen: *Off. Internat. du Vin Bul.,* November, 1930.

5. Mullin, F. J., N. Kleitman, and N. R. Cooperman: *Am. J. Physiol.,* **106**:478–487 (1933).

6. Masserman, J. H., and L. Jacobson: *Arch. Neurol. & Psychiat.*, **43**:334–340 (1940).

7. Billings: *Op. cit.* (p. 160).

8. Yorke-Davis, N. E.: *Wine and Health,* London, Chatto and Windus, 1909.

9. Ollier, L. F. A.: *Essai d'Oenologie Médicale,* Strasbourg Thèse ⚹466, 1859.

10. Eylaud and Macard: *Off. Internat. du Vin Bul.*, **6**:92 (1933).

11. Bonguiod, C.: *Considérations sur les Qualités et l'Usage du Vin,* Paris Thèse ⚹191, 1827.

12. Lozano, E. H.. *Rev. Vinicola y de Indust. Anex.*, **10**:17 (1939).

13. Vernon, H. M., et al.: *The Influence of Alcohol on Manual Work and Neuro-Muscular Co-ordination,* Medical Research Council Special Report ⚹34, 1919.

14. Billings: *Op. cit.* (p. 145).

15. a) Carpenter, T. M.: *J. Pharmacol. & Exper. Therap.*, **37**: 217–259 (1929).

   b) Canzanelli, A., R. Guild, and D. Rapport: *Am. J. Physiol.*, **110**:416 (1934).

   c) Chaikoff, I. L., C. L. Connor, and G. R. Biskind: *Am. J. Path.*, **14**:101–110 (1938).

16. Billings: *Op. cit.* (p. 147).

17. Lombard, W. P.: *J. Physiol.*, **13**:50 (1892).

18. Destree, E.; quoted by Billings: *Op. cit.* (p. 151).

19. Schumberg; quoted by Billings: *Op. cit.* (p. 152).

20. Scheffer; quoted by Billings: *Op. cit.* (p. 152).

21. Cabot, R. C.: *Boston Med. & Surg. J.*, **149**:93–101 (1903).

22. Auguet, A.: *Bull. Soc. scient. d'hyg. aliment.*, **23**:1–26 (1935).

23. Jaillet, J.: *De l'Alcool,* Paris, Doin, 1884 (p. 82).

24. Mauriac, E.: *Le Vin au Point de Vue Médical,* Paris, Doin, 1903.

25. Fitch, W. E.: *Pediatrics,* **24**:107 (1912).

26. Loeper, Maurice, and J. Alquier: *Progr. méd., Paris,* **44**: 1725–1730 (1929).

27. Cuvier, F.: *Le Vin,* Paris Thèse ⚹200, 1932 (p. 75).

28. Cazalis, R.: *Off. Internat. du Vin, IVᵉ Congrès Nat. des Médecins Amis des Vins de France,* **10**:2 (1937).

29. Kitchiner, William: *Art of Invigorating and Prolonging Life*, London, Hurst, 1822 (p. 198).
30. Anstie, Francis E.: *On the Uses of Wine in Health and Disease*, London, Practitioner, 1877 (pp. 60–61).
31. a) Strauss, M. B.: *Am. J. M. Sc.*, **189**:378–382 (1935).
    b) Spies, T. D.: *J. A. M. A.*, **110**:419 (1938).
32. Minot, G. R., M. B. Strauss, and S. Cobb: *New England J. Med.*, **208**:1244–1249 (1933).
33. Askey, J. M.: *California & West. Med.*, **51**:294–296 (1939).
34. Campbell, A. C. P., and J. H. Biggart: *J. Path. & Bact.*, **48**:245–262 (1939).
35. Lowry, J. V., W. H. Sebrell, F. S. Daft, and L. L. Ashburn: *J. Nutrition*, **24**:73–83 (1942).
36. Anstie: *Op. cit.* (pp. 58, 71).
37. Eylaud: *Off. Internat. du Vin Bul.*, **6**:119 (1933).
38. Trapp, C. E., and P. G. Schube: *J. Nerv. & Ment. Dis.*, **85**:668 (1937).
39. Alexandre and Aparici: *Valor Terapeutico del Vino de Jerez.* Internat. Medical Congress, 14th, Madrid, 1903; C. R. Sec. de Thérapeutique.
40. Weissenbach, R. J.: *Hôpital*, **24**:80 (1936).
41. Fabing, H. D., and M. A. Zeligs: *J. A. M. A.*, **117**:332 (1941).
42. Loebenstein-Loebel, E.: *Traité sur l'Usage et les Effets des Vins*, Strasbourg, Levrault, 1817.

IX. The Use of Wine in Acute Infectious Diseases

1. Dougnac, F.: *Día méd.*, **14**:292–294 (1942).
2. Anstie, Francis: *On the Uses of Wines in Health and Disease*, London, Practitioner, 1877 (p. 43).
3. *Ibid.* (p. 44).
4. *Ibid.* (p. 46).
5. *Ibid.* (p. 51).
6. Shaw, Peter: *The Juice of the Grape*, London, H. K. Lewis & Co., Ltd., 1724.
7. Osler, Sir William; quoted by E. H. Williams: *M. Rec.*, **92**:666 (1917).

8. Himwich, H. E.: *J. A. M. A.,* **100**:651–654 (1933).
9. Fantus, Bernard: *J. A. M. A.,* **69**:12 (1917).
10. Soresi, A. L.: *M. Rec.,* **141**:435 (1935).
11. Royer-Collard, H. L.: *De l'Usage et de l'Abus des Boissons Fermentées,* Paris, Guyot, 1838.
12. Bricheteau, E.: *Rev. de thér. méd-chir.,* **10**:485 (1862).
13. Anstie: *Op. cit.* (p. 44).
14. Wetmore, C. A.: *Pacific M. J.,* **48**:596 (1905).
15. Mauriac, E.: *Défense du Vin au Triple Point de Vue Économique, Hygiénique et Thérapeutique,* Xe Int. Congrès d'Hygiène et de Démographie, Paris, 1900.
16. Dougnac, F.: *Le Vin aux Points de Vue Physico-Chimique, Physiologique, Hygiénique, Thérapeutique,* Delmas, Chapon, Gounouilhou, 1935.
17. Violle, H., and E. Rosé: *Bull. Acad. nat. méd.,* **111**:733–739 (1934).
18. Kling, A.: *Je Sais Tout,* **30**:631 (1934).
19. Remlinger, P., and J. Bailly: *Rev. d'hyg.,* **59**:365 (1937).
20. Dietze, Werner; quoted by *Wines and Vines,* January, 1937.
21. Wetmore, C. A.: *Pacific M. J.,* **49**:17 (1906).
22. Bioletti, F. T.; quoted by C. A. Wetmore: *Pacific M. J.,* **49**:17 (1906).
23. Beckers, René: *Wines and Vines,* p. 14, February, 1940.
24. McNaught, B., and G. N. Pierce, Jr.: *Am. J. Clin. Path.,* **9**:52 (1939).

X. The Use of Wine in Diabetes Mellitus

1. Zuntz, N., and A. Magnus-Levy: *Arch. f. d. ges. Physiol.,* **49**:438 (1891).
2. Atwater, W. O., and F. G. Benedict: *Mem. Nat. Acad. Sc.,* **8**:231 (1902).
3. Benedict, H., and B. Török: *Ztschr. f. klin. Med.,* **60**: 329 (1906).
4. Neubauer, O.: *München. med. Wchnschr.,* **53**:791 (1906).
5. Diner, J.: *M. Rec.,* **100**:275 (1921).
6. Gavrila, J., and T. Sparchez: *Compt. rend. Soc. de biol.,* **98**:65–66 (1928).

7. Kolta, E.: *Deut. Arch. klin. Med.,* **175**:376–380 (1933).
8. Soula, G., and Baisset: *II*ᵉ *Congrès Nat. des Médecins Amis des Vins de France,* p. 330 (1935).
9. Burge, W. E.: *Science,* 48:327 (1918).
10. Tennent, D. M.: *Quart. J. Alcohol,* **2**:271–276 (1941).
11. Wiley, H. W.: *M. Times,* 44:175 (1916).
12. Porter, W. H.: *New York M. J.,* **111**:579 (1920).
13. Southgate, H. W.: *Biochem. J.,* **19**:737 (1925).
14. Weissenbach, R. J., Gilbert-Dreyfus, and J. Lièvre: Supplement; *Off. Internat. du Vin Bul.,* **8**:2 (1935).
15. Horder, T.: *Practitioner,* **113**:292 (1924).
16. Joslin, E. P., et al.: *The Treatment of Diabetes Mellitus,* Philadelphia, Lea & Febiger, 1952 (p. 230).
17. Mellanby, E.: *Brit. M. J.,* **2**:195 (1922).
18. Leary, Timothy: *New England J. Med.,* **205**:231–242 (1931).
19. Williamson, R. T.: *Diabetes Mellitus,* New York, The Macmillan Co., 1898.
20. Bridges, M. A.: *Dietetics for the Clinician,* Philadelphia, Lea & Febiger, 1941 (p. 862).
21. Weissenbach, Gilbert-Dreyfus, and Lièvre: *Op. cit.*
22. Dale, H. H., et al.: *Proc. Roy. Soc. Med., Sec. Therap. and Pharmacol.,* **13**:51 (1920).
23. Weissenbach, Gilbert-Dreyfus, and Lièvre: *Op. cit.*
24. Lepine, R.: *Le Diabète Sucré,* Paris, Baillière, 1909 (p. 677).
25. Jager, J.: *Le Valeur Alimentaire et Thérapeutique du Vin,* Paris Thèse ⚡550, 1938.
26. Weinstein, J. J., and J. H. Roe: *J. Lab. & Clin. Med.,* **40**:39 (1952).

XI. WINE AS A VEHICLE FOR MEDICATION

1. McKinley, A. P.: *Quart. J. Alcohol,* **11**:230–246 (1950).
2. Theophrastus: *Enquiry into Plants* (Loeb Classical Library), New York, G. P. Putnam's Sons, 1916.
3. Mnesitheus; quoted by McKinlay: *Op. cit.*
4. Pliny: *Natural History.* Bohn Classical Library, London, 1855.

5. Columella, L. J. M.: *On Agriculture* (Loeb Classical Library), Cambridge, Harvard University Press, 1941.
6. Celsus, A. C.: *De Medicina* (Loeb Classical Library), Cambridge, Harvard University Press, 1935.
7. Jager, J.: *La Valeur Alimentaire et Thérapeutique du Vin,* Paris Thèse ℳ550, 1938.
8. Fabing, H. D., and M. A. Zeligs: *J. A. M. A.,* **117**:332–334 (1941).
9. Neal, J. B., and S. M. Dillenberg: *New York State J. Med.,* **40**:1300–1302 (1940).
10. Fabing and Zeligs: *Op. cit.*
11. Gottschalk, A.: *Produits Pharm.,* **2**:376 (1947).

XII. The Use of Wine in the Treatment of the Aged and the Convalescent

1. Gardeton, C.: *Dictionnaire des Alimens,* Paris, Naudin, 1828 (p. 337).
2. Gaubert, P.: *Étude sur les Vins et les Conserves,* Paris, Mme. Crossant, 1857 (p. 250).
3. Thewlis, M. W.: *Care of the Aged* (*Geriatrics*), 4th Ed., St. Louis, C. V. Mosby Co., 1942 (p. 14).
4. *Ibid.*
5. Bonfort's Wine and Spirit Circular, **41**:260 (1894).
6. Thewlis: *Op. cit.* (p. 144).
7. Haggard, H. W., and E. M. Jellinek: *Alcohol Explored,* New York, Doubleday, Doran & Co., 1942 (p. 107).
8. Anstie, Francis: *On the Uses of Wine in Health and Disease,* London, Practitioner, 1877.
9. Salter, William T.: *Geriatrics,* **7**:317 (1952).
10. Brooks, Harlow: *Med. J. and Rec.,* **127**:201 (1928).
11. *Ibid.*
12. Stieglitz, E. J.: *J. A. M. A.,* **142**:1070–1077 (1950).
13. Leary, Timothy: *New England J. Med.,* **205**:231–242 (1931).
14. Loebenstein-Loebel, E.: *Traité sur l'Usage et les Effets des Vins,* Strasbourg, Levrault, 1817 (p. 100).
15. Bowes, A. de P., and C. F. Church: *Food Values of Portions*

Commonly Used, Philadelphia, Philadelphia Child Health Society, 1944 (p. 34).

16. Einhorn, Max; quoted by Harlow Brooks: *Med. J. and Rec.,* **127**:199–201 (1928).
17. Thewlis: *Op. cit.* (p. 144).
18. Hutchison, Robert: *Brit. J. Phys. Med.,* **9**:59 (1934).
19. Jackson, George H.: *The Medicinal Value of French Brandy,* Montreal, Thérien Frères, 1928 (pp. 245–246).
20. Adler, H. F., J. M. Beazell, A. J. Atkinson, and A. C. Ivy: *Quart. J. Alcohol,* **1**:638–644 (1941).
21. Leipoldt, C. Louis: *Wine and Spirit,* Stellenbosch, xi, No. 133, October, 1942.
22. Shaw, Peter: *Juice of the Grape,* London, H. K. Lewis & Co. Ltd., 1724 (p. 10).
23. Hitchcock, Edward: *Dyspepsia Forestalled and Resisted,* Amherst, Adams, 1831 (p. 30).
24. Barry, Edward: *Observations . . . on the Wines of the Ancients,* London, Cadell, 1775 (p. 42).
25. Pearl, R.: *Scient. Monthly,* **46**:462–483 (1938).
26. Billings, J. S., et al.: *Physiological Aspects of the Liquor Problem,* Vol. 1, New York, Houghton Mifflin Co., 1903 (p. 321).
27. Fabre, J. R.: *J. de méd. de Bordeaux,* **117**:509 (1940).
28. Sorel, R.: Abstract; *Off. Internat. du Vin Bul.,* **23**:83 (1950).
29. Farquharson, Robert; quoted by C. A. Rosewater: *J. M. Soc. New Jersey,* **16**:280 (1919).
30. Royer-Collard, H. L.: *De l'Usage et l'Abus des Boissons Fermentées,* Paris, Guyot, 1838.
31. Ollier, L. F. A.: *Essai d'Oenologie Médicale,* Strasbourg Thèse №466, 1859.
32. Pousson: *Off. Internat. du Vin Bul.,* **4**:31 (1931).
33. Dale, H. H., and others: *Proc. Roy. Soc. Med.,* Sec. Therap. and Pharmacol., **13**:47 (1920).
34. Bégin, M. E.: *L'Union Médicale,* 3rd ser., **20**:41 (1875).
35. Dale: *Op. cit.*
36. Pousson: *Op. cit.*
37. Greengard, Louis: *Fruit Prod. J.,* **20**:348 (1941).

XIII. The Elixir of the Grape

1. Saintsbury, George: *Notes on a Cellar Book,* New York, The Macmillan Co., 1933 (p. 34).
2. Allen, H. Warner: *The Romance of Wine,* New York, E. P. Dutton & Co., Inc., 1932 (p. 164).
3. Pavy, F. W.: *Treatise on Food and Dietetics,* Philadelphia, Lea, 1874 (p. 387).
4. Tovey, Charles: *Wine and Wine Countries,* London, Hamilton Adams & Co., 1862 (p. 288).
5. Anstie, Francis E.: *On the Uses of Wines in Health and Disease,* London, Practitioner, 1877 (p. 73).
6. Mistal, O.-M.: *Le Vin et le Jus de Raisin dans la Diététique et le Traitement des Affections Gastro-Intestinales chez les Tuberculeux.* IVe Congrès Nat. des Médecins Amis des Vins de France, 1937 (p. 71).
7. Berry, C. W.: *A Miscellany of Wine,* New York, Alfred A. Knopf, Inc., 1932 (p. 80).
8. Anstie: *Op. cit.* (p. 37).
9. *Ibid.* (p. 38).
10. Lucia, S. P.: *The Elixir of the Grape,* Lecture reprinted in *Harper's Wine and Spirit Gazette,* December 27, 1946 (p. 1009).
11. Tovey: *Op. cit.* (p. 93).
12. *Ibid.* (pp. 295–296).
13. Anstie: *Op. cit.* (p. 34).
14. Valaer, Peter: *Wines of the World,* New York, Abelard Press, Inc., 1950 (p. 56).
15. Druitt, Dr. Robert: *Report on the Cheap Wines from France, Germany, Italy, Austria, Greece, Hungary, and Australia: Their Use in Diet and Medicine,* London, Henry Renshaw, 1873 (p. 172).
16. Anstie: *Op. cit.* (p. 45).
17. *Ibid.* (p. 59).
18. Allen, H. Warner: *Sherry,* London, Constable's Wine Library, 1933 (p. 92).
19. Druitt: *Op. cit.* (p. 172).

20. Sandford, William: *A Few Practical Remarks on the Medicinal Effects of Wine and Spirits,* London, J. Tymbs, 1799 (p. 27).

21. Berry: *Op. cit.* (p. 94).

22. Allen: Sherry, *Op. cit.* (p. 92).

23. Anonymous: *Observations Concerning the Medical Virtues of Wine in a Letter to Dr. Buchan, late 1785, by a Gentleman of the Faculty,* London, Stuart and Stevenson, 1786 (pp. 11–15).

Index

‖‖